PRAI!
THE SECRET LANGU.
HOW TO ASK FOR THE CARE YOU DESERVE

M000222231

"This is a must-read book for anyone who is navigating the healthcare system. In my experience as a rheumatologist, I have seen patients struggle with decision-making around diagnosis, treatment and how to manage life in the face of serious illness. Robin Shapiro's personal narrative and those of her collaborators highlight important topics on aging, misdiagnosis, the impact of illness and errors of a sometimes faceless healthcare system. The magic in this book is easy-to-read, personal stories connecting us to why it is important to understand these topics along with simple steps we can take to be more effective when we seek care."

Steven S. Overman, MD MPH
Professor of Clinical Medicine, University of Washington
Co-author, *You Don't LOOK Sick: Living Well with Invisible Chronic Illness*

"Helping navigate this medical environment is challenging, increasing anxiety, which increases pain. Our main role as physicians, is helping people feel safe. This book is a remarkably clear and helpful resource, that should be a powerful guide to help people understand how they approach their medical choices."

David Hanscom, MD
Orthopedic Spine Surgeon (Retired)
Founder, Vertus, Inc.
Author, *Back in Control: A Surgeon's Roadmap Out of Chronic Pain*

"*The Secret Language of Healthcare* provides a valuable roadmap for any patient or family member who wants to take charge of their health. While our understanding and the field of health advocacy is really just starting, there is no doubt that patients need trusted, direct help. In this book, real-life medical scenarios are followed by key takeaways and practical tools to improve patient communication. Having survived medical errors in the hospital myself and as founder of a national directory of independent patient advocates, I believe this book and efforts to educate and empower patients are critical to improving our health – our very lives may depend on it!"

L. Bradley Schwartz, Esq.
President, Greater National Advocates

"You can't predict your circumstances or the future. But you can prepare. *The Secret Language of Healthcare* can help put you in a position to make the critical right choices. The "Why it Matters" sections of each chapter are especially valuable because they provide insights that can be used in diverse situations. The stories within the *The Secret Language of Healthcare* also expose why everyone should have an advocate when navigating the labyrinthine healthcare system. Your advocate doesn't always need to be a professional paid guide, but many times, that's your best bet."

Gordon Heinrichs, DC
Author, *Did Your Doctor Pass Communications 101?: How Miscommunication Endangers Your Life*

"When you face critical medical issues, time is of the essence, such as with a brain cancer diagnosis. *The Secret Language of Healthcare* shows us what to know and do in simple terms that anyone can understand. The power of this book is in the memorable stories and direct advice, including questions to ask and trusted resources to turn to. On a personal level and for the guidance that I can put into practice right now, the chapters on *Dementia* and *When to Fire the Doctor* spoke directly to me. This book is a gift to people who are struggling with the complexity of navigating health – a needed resource for everyone!"

Dellann Elliott Mydland,
President & Chair, EndBrainCancer Initiative

"In our organization, aging creatively speaks to how we can engage with our community and discover what it means to practice interdependence. Dealing with the increasingly confusing health care system requires new tools and strategies for interacting with doctors, hospitals and other care providers. This accessible and important book gives us resources, tools and real words to use as we relate to the health care system. It should be on hand for those of us who are aging and for the people who are committed to help us age well."

Rebecca Crichton
Executive Director, Northwest Center for Creative Aging

The

SECRET
LANGUAGE
of **HEALTHCARE**

HOW TO ASK FOR
THE CARE YOU DESERVE

The

SECRET
LANGUAGE
of **HEALTHCARE**

HOW TO ASK FOR
THE CARE YOU DESERVE

ROBIN L SHAPIRO

The Secret Language of Healthcare, Vol 1
Seattle WA
2019

Simpler Health Press
Seattle, WA
www.simplerhealth.press

ISBN: 978-1-7339666-0-3 (Print)
ISBN: 978-1-7339666-1-0 (E-book)

The names and stories in this book have been used with permission. Certain people have chosen to share their stories but wish to remain anonymous, in which case the author has selected a pseudonym to make their story easier to understand.

Profits from this book are intended to be distributed to not-for-profit organizations that support health advocacy efforts, including the Washington State Health Advocacy Association (WASHAA). For more information, visit www.washaa.org.

DISCLAIMER

Nothing in this book is intended to or provides any form of medical advice, counsel, treatment recommendation, or medical diagnoses, and shall not serve as a substitute under any circumstances for consulting with your own healthcare provider. The material provided in this book is designed to provide helpful information on the subjects discussed. The publisher, author, their agents and representatives are not responsible for any specific health or allergic conditions that may require medical supervision and are not liable for any damages or negative consequences from any treatment, action, application or preparation, to any person reading or following the information in this book. References are provided for informational purposes only and do not constitute an endorsement or validation of any information contained in any websites or other sources. Readers should know that the websites and links presented in this book reflect information posted as of the date accessed and noted in the reference links.

Please note that the opinions and views shared belong to the author and are not the opinions or views of any organization or company associated with the author.

DEDICATION

I dedicate this book to Beth Droppert, RN, BSN, a pioneer in the field of independent health advocacy.

ACKNOWLEDGEMENTS

Although I have always wanted to write a book, this book was conceived as a result of my conversations with Gordon Heinrichs and Beth Droppert in 2017. Gordon's original idea was to write a book on health literacy. We all knew that the goal of educating ordinary people on myriad subjects related to navigating health was important and urgent. I am grateful to Beth for bringing me into the world of independent health advocacy with her idea to start Allied Health Advocates, which we co-founded in 2008.

After a career working in health communications, public affairs, and biotechnology, I am appreciative to have met and worked with hundreds of patients over my 30+ years of working in healthcare. It is these stories that sparked the founding of my first company, Health Advocacy Strategies, in 2002.

I am grateful to business partner Cheryl Lubbert who joined me at Health Advocacy Strategies in 2010 and has been the driving force behind growing this original company to provide more patients with opportunities to share their stories having a positive impact on the healthcare of others.

Thank you to the original co-founders of WASHAA, Beth Droppert and Io Dolka, who remain committed to giving all patients access to insights and supports to make their health better. I also feel fortunate to work with an outstanding Board.

Thanks go to all the contributors to this book for so generously spending the time allowing me to interview them and share their wisdom.

To my friends who are fellow writers, Doug Levy, Lana Lauher Guernsey, Cynthia Hartwig, Anne-Frans Van Vliet and Mel Zakaluk, thanks for giving me great feedback and for being such a constant, positive impact in my life. I also am grateful to Alicia Dunams and her team who helped make this book possible.

Last, but not least, I would like to thank my family. My father encouraged me early in life to think big and work hard. While he died of glioblastoma (brain cancer) in 2008, I am fortunate to feel his spirit alongside of me. Thank you to my mom who has always been amazed by the human body and served as our family's Dr. Mom. I am grateful for the support of my children and most of all, my husband, Mike, who has always been 100% unwavering in his belief in me in all things. The greatest gift I have in the world is the love of my family and friends.

FOREWORD

In my more than 40-year career as a nurse and health advocate leader, I have been passionate about educating the public about the importance of being prepared. But it wasn't until my own, personal experience with a brain tumor that I understood the urgency and the gaps in the healthcare system from such a personal perspective.

As past President of the Case Management Society of America, Founder of the Professional Patient Institute, and Governor for District 27 of Quota International, I have been on the frontlines of this emerging field of independent health advocates, which is how I know Robin Shapiro. I have been involved in the development of training and credentials for multiple types of health care professionals, including nurses, case managers and professional patient advocates. And I have always felt that patients need to be in the center of healthcare choices. Knowing what to say is key. However, it is hard to speak for yourself when you are sick.

Over the years, Robin and I have had many discussions about the importance of educating people to know how to be their own advocate. Her book, *The Secret Language of Healthcare: How to Ask for the Care You Deserve*, is a fitting continuation to the urgent work of educating the public about the significant risks of not understanding the healthcare system. Her practical tips and language suggestions are both simple and specific.

Given my significant experience as a critical care and case management nurse, I thought I knew how healthcare worked. I had confidence that I could advocate for myself and manage my own care. All that changed in 2014 after I was involved in a minor car accident. As a result, I could not drive home, so I called my husband Corky. When he arrived, I told him what happened, and he looked me over as well as my vehicle. Despite feeling okay and just wanting to go home, he insisted we go to the hospital.

We went to a small hospital emergency room in our neighborhood where I was evaluated by the emergency department physician. After his assessment, he ordered a CAT scan. Once back, the doctor sat with Corky and me and told us that I had a brain tumor. He would have to admit me to the hospital for an evaluation by a neurologist and a neurosurgeon. I don't recall much after that initial conversation. Blanks have been filled in by my husband and a few friends, but I knew in that instant my life had changed.

Because I was the patient, my husband stepped in and spoke for me. He asked questions and made decisions. In addition to calling our family members to let them know what was happening, he called two friends and asked for help. One was a longtime friend and nurse case manager colleague, Marilyn Van Houten and the other was a patient advocate, Cathy Bowers. Both came to the hospital and talked to the neurosurgeon about my plan of care. After hearing the diagnosis and the plan of care, they asked my husband if they could work to get me to a major teaching hospital in my area, where I could be treated by specialists. They also gave him tips on what to look for, the importance of keeping notes on what was happening and most importantly to be present, so I was safe and taken care of.

After I was transferred to the teaching hospital, a brain biopsy was performed which led to the diagnosis of a central nervous system lymphoma. I was referred to a hematologist who specialized in this type of tumor. After evaluating me, he prescribed aggressive treatment which I started immediately. Today, I am glad to say I am tumor free.

Looking back on my experience proved several things to me: First, everyone needs an advocate. You should not go into the healthcare system alone. I was lucky that my husband could advocate for me. I also had my friends Marilyn and Cathy who helped him understand the system and gave him ideas on alternatives to the current plan of care.

Second, we had prepared for this emergency by talking to each other about what each of us would want if we were not able to speak for ourselves, before something happened. Corky knew my wishes, and I knew his.

What this experience taught me more than anything is that you need to know what to ask for when you are thrust into the healthcare system.

Unfortunately, the healthcare system is complex, fragmented, and has a language of its own, so it is challenging for users to understand how it works and what choices we have. If we are honest, most of us don't think about our healthcare until it is threatened. It is not easy to be a patient, but with education, support, communication, and collaboration among all members of the team, we can turn the tide.

As the healthcare industry transforms to a more patient-centered system, *YOU* will need to be more involved, ask questions, and do the research that needs to be done to take care of your health. It is up to you, with the help of the healthcare team to chart your journey.

That is why *The Secret Language of Healthcare: How to Ask for the Care You Deserve* is a must read. This book will open your eyes to the complexity of the healthcare system and the role each of us plays when we are thrust into the system. It might not be you, but your wife, husband, child, sister, or brother, so we all need to be prepared. This book will give you insights into the challenges you may face and how best to handle them.

Be the one in your family to start the conversation. What does each member of your family want to happen if they become sick or injured? Don't wait till there is a crisis, as you never know when your life will change – this book will help you and your loved ones be prepared!

Anne Llewellyn, MS, BHSA, RN-BC, CCM, CRRN
Nurse Advocate Digital Blogger at nursesadvocates.com

TABLE OF CONTENTS

INTRODUCTION

THE PROBLEM

Most Americans do not think a lot about being prepared to navigate the healthcare system and overlook that at our peril:

- The third leading cause of death in America is people dying from preventable medical events in the hospital. Heart disease and cancer are the top two reasons how people die in our country.[1]

- Most people spend more time researching a car purchase than they do researching their doctor or hospital, according to a 2012 Harris Interactive poll, released by Healthgrades.

Healthcare is complicated. And no one wants to be a patient, so when we face a healthcare challenge, we are ill-equipped to understand how the healthcare system works. Most of the language used by health professionals is very complicated and unknown to ordinary people. That is why it is always helpful to have a doctor or nurse in the family. If you do, you have a leg up because they speak the same language.

---

[1] *BMJ* 2016; 353:i2139

THE SOLUTION

People who are more active in their healthcare have better healthcare outcomes (results) and lower healthcare costs.[2] So how do we do it?

We need to find a way to help people become more confident and competent in navigating healthcare. I wrote this book to focus on translating keywords and phrases that can help any ordinary person find better care. It is the hidden language of healthcare that is preventing everyday people from understanding what to do and how to talk to healthcare providers so we may be effective in getting the care we all want and deserve.

MY PERSPECTIVE

Unlocking this hidden language in healthcare is key based on my 30+ years working in the health field, primarily in roles that focused on understanding patient stories. I started my career working with the federal government's public education campaign in the 1980s, called America Responds to AIDS. In 1987, Americans believed that AIDS was the most urgent health issue in our country, according to a Gallup poll.[3] My first work assignment was to contribute to the landmark mailing from Surgeon General C. Everett Koop to every household in America. The brochure was called Understanding AIDS.[4]

As communications director at biotechnology company, Immunex Corporation, my favorite part of the job was working with and responding to patients. In fact, a patient from Spokane, WA would be the touchstone for my work there and the inspiration for founding my first company in 2002, called Health Advocacy Strategies.

---

[2] HEALTH AFFAIRS 34, NO. 3 (2015): 431–437
[3] https://news.gallup.com/poll/4324/aids-issue-fades-among-americans.aspx
[4] HHS Publication No. (CDC) HHS-88-8404

Kerry contacted Immunex in the late 1990s, explaining that she had been an active teen, involved in every sport imaginable until rheumatoid arthritis crippled her hands and feet. Despite these limitations she had married and had a baby. Although her rheumatoid arthritis went into remission during her pregnancy, it raged after her baby was born, preventing her from being able to use her hands. Kerry told me she had to diaper her baby with her teeth. With the medicine that Immunex made, her disease symptoms diminished substantially, helping her to use her hands and be fully engaged in her life. Kerry had wanted to thank the creators of the medicine, but also to make sure other patients could understand that even in dire medical situations there is reason to have hope. Patient stories like Kerry's, of overcoming life-limiting disease symptoms, continue to inspire me.

This work led me to found companies that could help patients find their voices to help others who face similar health situations. In 2007, I met Beth Droppert, RN, BSN and co-founded Allied Health Advocates soon after – the first state-wide, independent health advocate company in Washington state, where our nurse and insurance advocates could be hired directly by patients and their families to help navigate healthcare.

We found that few people knew what health advocacy was or why it was needed. So, Beth, Io Dolka, and I co-founded the Washington State Health Advocacy Association (WASHAA), to help increase awareness about what health advocacy is, to help teach people skills, and connect people to health advocacy resources (professionals, education, organizations) to help get better care.

It is through the last two decades doing this work that I have received a first-hand look at what happens when ordinary people try to navigate the very complicated healthcare system. Through WASHAA, I have worked with others to create presentations, training, and materials that provide this learning to the public.

I am passionate about this topic because:

- Most people know what to do in their health situation *only after* they have already been through their experience.
- There is considerable room for improvement in the patient experience — the result of which might be fewer deaths and fewer unnecessary side effects.
- The data is clear; more active and engaged patients mean better health and lower costs.
- We created a lot of content through our years working in this field, and people need to know these concepts.

THE BENEFITS OF READING THIS BOOK

By reading this book, you will be able to:

- easily understand some common language and concepts to look for when hospitalized, when working with your doctor, or when facing a medical diagnosis
- immediately put the concepts to use by reading about when to use suggested statements and questions
- practice the way to use words or phrases of the medical profession by reading examples
- look up additional reading materials if you are curious about the data behind the concept

CAN WE MAKE HEALTH CARE SIMPLER?

I wrote this book for anyone who wants to be more involved in their healthcare but might not know exactly how. Through unforgettable stories and step-by-step guides for how to use recommended language, you will gain confidence in your ability to navigate healthcare more effectively.

Don't wait to read this! Most of these chapters contain potentially life-saving wisdom from a wide variety of people who have lived through serious medical situations. It is my hope you will read this book, share it with those you love (or even buy a copy for all those you love) so you all can have it close at hand when you need it.

I would love to know what you think. What was most powerful? Most actionable? What do you think is missing? Please contact me at: Robin@Robin-Shapiro.Com. I would love to hear from you!

To your good health,
Robin

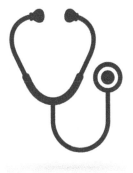

SECTION 1

IT CAN HAPPEN
TO ANYONE

SECTION 1

IT CAN HAPPEN TO ANYONE

When I was growing up in St. Louis, Missouri, I had no reference for medical situations. I am the daughter of an entrepreneur father and artist/stay-at-home mom. My mom inspired me to be curious and in awe of the human body. My father was all about work — working hard in order to learn and do things well.

Although I always had an interest in health and healthcare, it wasn't until I started to work with patients and heard their stories that I began to think about the randomness of people needing to interact with the healthcare system. People do not expect to be working with doctors. We cannot say that a particular person will develop rheumatoid arthritis, for instance. No one expects to be in a life-changing car accident or experience common side effects that happen in hospitals.

There is no standard preparation for being a patient. There should be some basic common knowledge that everyone has. I hope that the chapters in this section will inspire you to learn more!

FOR FURTHER LEARNING:

- ✓ Attend or host a ***Patient Know More!*** presentation by a WASHAA representative: http://www.washaa.org/request-a-presentation.html.
- ✓ Order and play The Hello Game: https://commonpractice.com/products/hello-game. Provocative questions in a game format walk you through discussions about what matters most to you.

ACTION ITEMS:

- ✓ Fill out an advance directive that tells those you love what you want should you not be able to choose for yourself.
- ✓ Have a conversation with your loved ones about what matters to you.
- ✓ Make sure you have a will, and tell people where it is, or provide them with a copy.
- ✓ Select a healthcare proxy. This is the person who will be your decision-maker for healthcare if you are unable to express your wishes.

You will discover specific resources by reading the chapters in this section. Just remember, we might not be able to control what happens to us, but we can be prepared to give ourselves the best experience possible when we navigate the healthcare system.

CHAPTER 1

FIRST, BRUSH MY TEETH: KNOW WHAT TO ASK FOR

It was 2010, a few years after we started the first independent health advocacy company in Washington state, Allied Health Advocates, when the phone rang with a story I will never forget. Ted wanted to hire a health advocate for his wife who had been in the hospital for a year, in a coma for at least part of the time. He had just heard that the hospital wanted to pull all of her teeth. What was remarkable was that prior to going into the hospital, she had just had all of her teeth re-capped and they were in perfect condition. Ted told me that when he had asked the hospital if they had seen issues when they brushed her teeth, the hospital replied that they had not brushed her teeth – ever. This was a memorable story for me.

This story made me wonder how something so basic, so essential to self-care, could be overlooked. Although I never spoke with the hospital, it was a powerful image that stuck with me.

Seven years later, my good friend Deborah's husband, Reid, was in the hospital to address nutrition and pain issues related to his prostate cancer. Reid was a quiet, tall (over 6 feet) long-time engineer for Boeing, with a gentle, kind spirit and loved taking landscape photos. Although I didn't know Reid well, I always admired his positive attitude and his ready-for-anything relationship with Deborah. He always focused on what was going well.

I visited Reid in the hospital before his meeting with an attorney who would arrive later in the day. It was to be the main effort for his day, as Reid was growing increasingly weak. I asked him how he wanted to prepare for his meeting with the attorney. After giving it some thought, he said he would like to shave and be dressed in his clothes instead of the hospital gown. By this point, he had been in the hospital for four days. Although a typical hospital stay would include a shower every couple of days, I learned that sometimes that doesn't happen unless someone asks. Although he could walk with help and was awake much of his hospital stay, he was fairly weak, but still had a very strong spirit. Reid was too weak to shower or shave on his own. He could lift a spoon to his mouth with significant effort. I asked about whether he had brushed his teeth and he quietly said "no." I asked if he would like his teeth brushed. Although he couldn't speak clearly, he nodded his head vigorously. It had been four days since someone brushed his teeth.

When asked, the nurse took care of brushing his teeth right away, giving Reid the dignity and confidence he deserved. It was a little but important thing. But you had to know to ask.

WHY IT MATTERS:

- Preventative oral care lowers overall costs in the long run, so take care of your teeth before it is an issue.[5]

---

[5] http://ajph.aphapublications.org/doi/abs/10.2105/AJPH.2009.184747

- Lack of oral care in the hospital can lead to other health issues, such as pneumonia if a person is on a ventilator.[6] In fact, being on a ventilator is a key risk factor in hospital-acquired pneumonia. One study found that increased assessment, cleaning, and suctioning of non-ventilator patients reduced hospital acquired pneumonia by 37%.[7]

- After staying in the hospital for a day or two, bacteria in your mouth become more like the hospital environment. Bacteria replicates so quickly in your mouth that it can take only a matter of hours to cause problems.[8]

USING THIS INFORMATION:

1. When hospitalized, ask the nursing staff how they handle oral health, including teeth brushing. How will they handle your loved one's mouth care?

2. Be prepared to help if needed.

3. Certain diseases and treatments can cause sores in the mouth, which might require mouth rinses or swabbing instead of teeth brushing. Sometimes patients may have trouble swallowing.

4. When a patient is on a ventilator, it is particularly important that mouth rinses or swabbing are used to cleanse the mouth.

---

[6] http://www.strategiesfornursemanagers.com/content.cfm?content_id=229444&oc_id=602#

[7] https://www.beckershospitalreview.com/quality/non-ventilator-hospital-acquired-pneumonia-are-you-addressing-the-hidden-issue-affecting-more-patients-at-a-greater-cost-than-vap.html

[8] https://sacramentodentistry.com/oral-health/expecting-a-hospital-stay-pack-your-toothbrush/

SPECIFIC LANGUAGE YOU CAN USE:

- I am wondering how the hospital typically handles oral health for patients.
- Could you share with us how the nursing staff intends to handle oral health with our case?
- What can I do to help with oral care while we are here?

ADDITIONAL READING AND RESOURCES:

- To find a free or low-cost sliding scale dental clinic in your area: http://www.needymeds.org/dental-clinics
- The Joint Commission urges enforcement of oral care policies: https://www.hcpro.com/ACC-328832-4634/Joint-Commission-urges-enforcement-of-oral-care-policies.html
- *Teeth*, by Mary Otto: A book showing how oral health influences all aspects of our lives: https://www.amazon.com/Teeth-Beauty-Inequality-Struggle-America/dp/1620971445

ABOUT THE CONTRIBUTOR:

Deborah Wakefield has shared her husband, Reid's, story and it is used with permission.

CHAPTER 2

STROKE: KNOW THE SYMPTOMS

During my career, I have been blessed to know many driven health communications professionals, including Stacie Byars. Like me, she loved to work, and it was always a central part of her life. But at 51, she suffered from a stroke that changed her life. Stacie was an unlikely candidate for stroke, having never had high cholesterol or high blood pressure. Although she considers herself lucky, she would like others to learn from her experience and hopefully prevent a more serious health crisis by not getting help fast enough.

On the morning of Monday, April 18, 2016, Stacie was going for a run in her hilly neighborhood of Mukilteo outside Seattle, WA. The Friday before she had returned from an international trip to Copenhagen and, though jet-lagged, had worked throughout the weekend on a big photoshoot that was to take place in California. She had recently ramped up her already heavy work schedule, launching her own communications consulting business. She was feeling tired and thought a run might help before she flew to California that day.

On her run downhill, three and a half miles to the water, she felt her right eye go cloudy, which she chalked up to being fatigued. She didn't know that a common symptom of stroke is to have problems in one or both eyes. This was her first symptom, which she knew occurred at 10 a.m., because she always clocked her runs. Since she couldn't see well, she decided to cut her run short and turn back up the hill. She felt unusually tired.

After a quick shower, she stubbed her toe on the shower edge and was frustrated because it really hurt, and she was in a hurry to pack and catch her flight. She didn't realize this was the first sign that the left side of her body was developing weakness.

She finished packing and left for the airport. Just a mile away from her house, a car passed her and she didn't see it, causing a minor car accident. When she went to exchange information with the other driver, she couldn't quite remember what information she should be collecting. This was very out of character for her. She didn't know that this was another sign of stroke – memory lapse.

Stacie called her husband Dave to tell him about the accident and mentioned that she was really tired. He suggested that she get to bed early once in California. She was not slurring her speech, like many people who have a stroke, so Dave thought nothing about her fatigue.

On the flight to California, Stacie got her suitcase down from the overhead bin so she could work during the flight. But she couldn't lift her suitcase back up when it was time to stow it. She was a seasoned traveler, typically on the road about 200 days a year, with lots of international flights. She had never had any difficulty lifting her bag before. She asked a fellow passenger to help her with her bag and said, "just a little tired today." Upon her return from using the bathroom on the flight, she noticed she was staggering as she walked back down the aisle to her seat, but was too focused on the meeting the following day to give it much thought.

Stacie landed in California, took a taxi to the hotel, and called Dave before going to bed early. When she got up in the middle of the night to go to the bathroom, she fell to the floor. The entire left side of her body was paralyzed. Lying on the floor, she kicked the floor and screamed for help. The man in the room next door yelled for her to be quiet because it was 2:00 a.m., but Stacie eventually convinced him to contact the front desk. When a staff person came to the door, she asked if Stacie was on drugs or drunk. Stacie finally convinced her that something was terribly wrong and to contact the EMT. Eventually Stacie was taken by ambulance to the nearest hospital. The EMT told her that if the hospital had been farther away, she would have died from her stroke.

When Dave finally connected with the hospital, it was shift change and they did not have a lot of information – only that Stacie had a stroke, her vitals were strong, and she would never be the same. Dave was very anxious, not knowing what shape Stacie would be in when he would see her. He booked the next available flight.

Stacie told me that without her husband serving as her health advocate, she would have been in bad shape. She had no control of the left side of her body and was in the intensive care unit for six days. She had to use a bedpan which they would leave under her for long periods of time, which was uncomfortable and frustrating. After a week, she couldn't sit up, walk, or do much of anything, and certainly wasn't strong enough to fly home.

Stacie and Dave found a rehabilitation facility in California and Stacie moved there. She would be there for four weeks. Dave had slept on a futon at the hospital, but there was nowhere for him to stay at the rehabilitation facility. On the weekends, he would rent a hotel and a car. He worked during the week because they needed the income.

Financially, the stroke dramatically changed their lives. In the early weeks of recovery, the costs of travel alone were high. Stacie was no longer earning an income and she did not have any disability or long-term care insurance. The insurance coverage they had through Dave's job had a very high deductible. And right as she was being discharged from the rehabilitation facility, someone notified them that their huge bill for the ambulance was going to collections for non-payment. Stacie said that they were fortunate because they had saved money as dual income earners and didn't have kids, but the bills were daunting.

Stacie could use a wheelchair and eat with her right hand, but had lost her ability to make sound decisions. She had occupational therapy, physical therapy, and speech therapy six times a week. Stacie said that the rehab center was also a traumatic brain injury unit, so everyone around her had suffered a stroke, a car crash, or other unexpected brain injury. She felt very lucky that her losses were not as bad as others around her.

Stacie enjoyed going to the dining room and eating with people who were recovering. Being grateful was a core healing technique that helped her cope and slowly regain control of her life. Every day, as part of her therapy, Stacie would write her goals and keep a diary. As part of speech therapy, she would read her goals aloud from her diary the following day. Stacie said it was incredibly humbling, and she struggled emotionally about not being able to go back to work. But she also felt very lucky to be able to focus on her recovery. She loved to cook, so her husband researched assistive technology cooking tools might work for her. Stacie learned to hold a tool in her left hand and cook with her right hand.

When Stacie returned home, the downstairs bedroom became her living area. Dave built a ramp and she could use her wheelchair, but he could not leave her alone. They hired a caregiver to help Stacie at home while Dave was at work. The cost was $27 per hour, and Stacie said this was one of the most expensive aspects of her care. She continued to get occupational therapy, speech therapy, and physical therapy to help her walk. The caregiver would drive her to appointments. Stacie began to get stronger and eventually, she could take the bus everywhere, and friends rallied to help. She went to the

YMCA every day to exercise, and in September 2017 could take the written and driving test to get her driver's license reinstated.

Stacie's story is very inspiring. She says that surviving the stroke completely changed her life and redefined for her and Dave what it means to be lucky. She has learned to ask for help, too. She says she feels fortunate to be able to exercise, which includes going to spin class. The people there help her on her bike and make sure her feet are properly placed. She continues to cook and has more time to spend at home. Gratitude is a central focus in her life and has enabled Stacie to continue to live a full, rich life.

WHY IT MATTERS:

Stroke is the leading cause of disability in the United States, with approximately 795,000 people suffering a stroke each year.[9]

- A stroke happens when the brain's blood vessels are blocked or burst, denying the brain of the blood and oxygen it requires, causing brain cells to die.

- If you are having symptoms of a stroke, getting help fast is important to prevent brain damage. Getting help quickly can limit brain damage and serious side effects. If you arrive at the emergency room within three hours of your first symptoms, you might have less disability three months after the stroke than if your care is delayed.[10]

- The CDC notes these symptoms for stroke in men and women:
  - sudden numbness or weakness in the face, arm, or leg, especially on one side of the body

---

[9] http://www.strokecenter.org/patients/about-stroke/stroke-statistics/
[10] Fang J, Keenan NL, Ayala C, Dai S, Merritt R, Denny CH. Awareness of stroke warning symptoms—13 states and the District of Columbia, 2005. MMWR 2008;57:481–5.

○ sudden confusion, trouble speaking, or difficulty understanding speech

○ sudden trouble seeing in one or both eyes

○ sudden trouble walking, dizziness, loss of balance, or lack of coordination

○ sudden severe headache with no known cause

USING THIS INFORMATION:

1. Stacie recommends that people pay attention to their body. When you don't feel well, don't ignore symptoms that can be indicators of a serious problem.

2. The Centers for Disease Control and Prevention (CDC) recommends that you note the time when any symptoms first appear. This information helps healthcare providers determine the best treatment for each person. Do not drive to the hospital or let someone else drive you. Call an ambulance so that medical personnel can begin life-saving treatment on the way to the emergency room.

3. Some people are at greater risk for stroke. If you smoke, are obese, have high blood pressure, high cholesterol or diabetes, you are at higher risk.[11]

4. If you are African American or Hispanic, you might be at greater risk. See the additional reading and resources below.

---

[11] Benjamin EJ, Blaha MJ, Chiuve SE, et al. on behalf of the American Heart Association Statistics Committee and Stroke Statistics Subcommittee. Heart disease and stroke statistics—2017 update: a report from the American Heart Association. Circulation. 2017;135:e229-e445.

5. According to the National Stroke Association, women may report symptoms that are different from the common symptoms. They include:

- loss of consciousness or fainting
- general weakness
- difficulty breathing or shortness of breath
- confusion, unresponsiveness or disorientation
- sudden behavioral change
- agitation
- hallucination
- nausea or vomiting
- pain
- seizures
- hiccups

SPECIFIC LANGUAGE YOU CAN USE:

Know the signs of stroke! The CDC uses the acronym FAST to remember the signs and symptoms:

- **F — Face:** "Smile for me." Does one side of the face droop?
- **A — Arms:** "Raise both of your arms." Does one arm drift downward?
- **S — Speech:** "Repeat after me. Breakfast is served at eight." Is their speech slurred or strange?
- **T — Time:** If you see any of these signs, call 911 right away. Time is of the essence in treatment.

ADDITIONAL READING AND RESOURCES:

To learn more about the different types of stroke, here is an overview from the Stroke Association: https://www.strokeassociation.org/en/about-stroke.

Useful facts sheets from the CDC[12]:

- Stroke
- Know the Facts About Stroke
- Know the Signs and Symptoms of Stroke
- Women and Stroke
- Men and Stroke
- African-American Women and Stroke
- African-American Men and Stroke
- Hispanic Women and Stroke—Las Mujeres Hispanas y Los Accidentes Cerebrovasculares
- Hispanic Men and Stroke—Los Hombres Hispanos y Los Accidentes Cerebrovasculares
- Hispanics and Stroke—Las Personas Hispanas y Los Accidentes Cerebrovasculares

---

[12] https://www.cdc.gov/stroke/facts.htm

CHAPTER 3

WHEN THE DIAGNOSIS IS DEMENTIA

We all know someone who is living with dementia or has a loved one who is. Two dear childhood friends are struggling to manage parents living afar. In each instance, their mothers are experiencing symptoms of dementia and their fathers are not really wanting to address it. This chapter is for all of us who are dealing with this dreaded disease – and provides a guide for what to do.

I first met Annie Jacobsen 10 years ago when she owned Assisted Transitions, a business that focused on helping seniors downsize their belongings and move to a smaller home. Annie's business now focuses on dementia, and I asked her to share a compelling story that would put into context the challenges that many people face with this diagnosis.

Kirk, an Arlington, WA stone sculptor, had been a client of Annie's in 2012 when he was in his 70s. Kirk's wife Judy was diagnosed 6–12 months prior and was in mid-stage dementia. Mid-stage dementia meant that she was at risk for wandering. She was often highly agitated, and caring for her in their large home with acreage was becoming increasingly difficult. During the time Annie was helping them prepare for a smaller home, she witnessed many of their dilemmas living with the disease.

Judy would become agitated when Kirk wasn't nearby. Many mornings she would wake up, roll over, grasp Kirk's hand and say, "I love you so much." He frequently mentioned how much this helped him start another day. It was increasingly difficult for Kirk to care for his wife because years of sculpting had left him with a bad back. Judy started to need help getting out of bed and needed all of her meals prepared for her. Kirk began to look physically exhausted and depleted. His shoulders were hunched, and he fretted about what to do in the face of potentially not being able to care for the love of his life.

Kirk and Judy knew that they should move, but Kirk was hesitant to do it. He joined a caregivers' support group, which was pivotal to helping him think through decisions, especially those around the sale of the house. When Judy started to need help showering, toileting, and doing more things that couldn't necessarily be planned in advance, he knew it was time to move. She began to forget how to stand and walk. When Kirk's brother visited from out of town, his observations as a supportive outsider helped it become clear that there was urgency to their move.

In Annie's experience it is important to make a move while the person experiencing dementia is in early to mid-stage cognitive change, so they still have some capacity to build new memories and gather new information. Learning new things through repetition (like walking to the dining hall or the general location of your room) is more likely when someone moves before reaching the later stages of dementia when it is difficult to learn new patterns.

Annie has seen how the disease affects a wide range of families, and says it seems that the decision to move a person living with dementia to memory care is always harder on the spouse or deciding family member. Feelings of guilt for "throwing in the towel," "taking the easy road" or "giving up" on your spouse or partner who is living with dementia can be very intense. It is important to have support.

Judy's disease took its toll on Kirk. He was diagnosed with prostate cancer while preparing for the move. Upon reflection, Kirk felt he waited six months too long to move Judy to a place that could provide her care. He was experiencing extreme anxiety and wasn't sleeping well. For periods lasting several hours or sometimes days, Judy didn't recognize Kirk, even though they had been married for 30 years, saying threateningly "when my husband gets home…."

One of the social workers who Kirk worked with advised, "You have moved beyond hired part-time home care assistance when the needs of your loved one are no longer schedulable." When your loved one needs help to toilet and perform typical activities of daily living, like walking and dressing, it is time to consider a move or to have 24-hour care. In the end, Kirk's own diagnosis urgently necessitated a move for Judy.

Annie suggests people consider these issues when evaluating what to do for someone with dementia:

- Seek an accurate diagnosis from a specialist (typically a gerontologist or neurologist) who will identify the stage of dementia.

- Evaluate if the well partner is receiving the support that he or she needs and the level of their physical or emotional suffering.

- Notice if details and timelines have begun to blur. Keep a journal to review what is happening over time. Sometimes you don't see what the challenges are day-to-day, but you can see a pattern of decreasing competence over time.

- Have a family conversation well before you think you need to, when everyone is healthy, to help understand what is important to family members (Refer to the resources below.). Many families say it puts their minds at ease knowing this difficult conversation is covered and they don't need to fret about it.

- In the early stage of dementia, appeal to your family member's interest to retain control and ask their opinion when you notice changes in behavior (See sample language below.).

Every family is different, and although we all wish there was a practical guide for when to move someone and what to do, a clear right choice is likely to be elusive. The decision is often prompted by a crisis with the primary caregiver. Ideally, a family can decide prior to a crisis, and this is where planning and a support network really help.

WHY IT MATTERS:

- About 5.7 million Americans have Alzheimer's dementia. By mid-century, the number of people living with Alzheimer's dementia in the United States is projected to grow to 13.8 million.[13]

- One in 10 people age 65 and older (10 percent) has Alzheimer's dementia. Almost two-thirds of Americans with Alzheimer's are women. One in three seniors dies with dementia.[14]

---

[13] https://www.alzheimersanddementia.com/article/S1552-5260(18)30041-4/abstract
[14] https://www.alz.org/alzheimers-dementia/facts-figures

- Dementia does not just happen to people who are older; it is estimated to affect about 200,000 people in the United States who are in their 40s and 50s.

- Although memory loss is the most recognized dementia symptom, other symptoms include: challenging and changing behaviors and moods, difficulty starting or completing a familiar task, or an inability to communicate or recognize loved ones.

USING THIS INFORMATION:

1. It is useful to make videos of people and family to use as time goes by. A client recently shared a story of a former surgeon with late stage dementia who loved watching and narrating surgeries found on youtube.com with his caregiver. It gave him great joy and he knew exactly what was happening in the surgery.

2. Engaging in music or movement classes is often enjoyable for people with dementia. Annie assisted in a ukulele class and although a recent client's family was skeptical their loved one would be interested because he was early stage dementia, he loved the class.

3. Families need to not focus on a tragedy narrative of the diagnosis, and instead, find ways to connect with loved ones through conversation, story-telling, and activities without expected outcomes. Here is a good article: https://www.washingtonpost.com/local/social-issues/changing-the-tragedy-narrative-why-a-growing-camp-is-promoting-a-joyful-approach-to-alzheimers/2019/02/21/2c4ed4f0-2244-11e9-81fd-b7b05d5bed90_story.html?noredirect=on&utm_term=.9fc07688b5e4

SPECIFIC LANGUAGE YOU CAN USE:

With Medical Providers

If you are seeing a general practitioner, ask to have your loved one who is living with dementia evaluated with a cognitive test. The MoCA is currently considered the best tool, as it can detect mild cognitive impairment. Other tests include: SLUMS, Mini-Cog and the MMSE/Mini-Mental. These are 10–15-minute tests that can measure if cognitive skills are declining over time. Here are some questions you can ask:

- What type of dementia is it?
- What is the stage or how far has it progressed?
- What can I expect in terms of changes I may experience, based on my individual diagnosis?
- What are my treatment options? What potential side effects will they pose?
- What are the best ways to address potential safety concerns? (confusion, wandering, driving)
- What symptoms and behaviors signal significant progression and need reassessment, or if it is time to call you?
- What resources do you recommend in our community?
- Are there any clinical trials or research studies that you recommend we consider?

For adult children trying to have a conversation with a parent with dementia or a well parent, Annie recommends stating what you observe and, in a non-judgmental way, ask about the changes you are observing:

- I noticed that the conversation about cousin Joe's wedding next month seemed to confuse you at dinner. Is this something that is happening more often? Have you been finding it hard to track other conversations lately?

- I've noticed (a) mail/bills stacking up, (b) the house doesn't seem as fresh as usual, (c) you have missed our weekly lunch date a few times, (d) the car has some new scratches. Are you noticing any differences, or are some tasks a bit more frustrating?

- Appeal to your loved one's desire to retain independence by bringing them into the conversation instead of talking at them, with these suggested phrases:

  - What is your opinion about what happened last night at dinner?

  - What do you think we should do about ensuring the bills are paid on time?

  - How are you feeling about shopping and cooking meals? Would you like me to help with this a few times during the week?

ADDITIONAL READING AND RESOURCES:

- Momentia is a Washington-based program about engagement for early stage dementia decline where people can still feel their personhood, and these resources can be used anywhere: http://www.momentiaseattle.org/programs

- The Alzheimer's Association has many resources, especially for identifying the stages of dementia, including: https://www.alz.org/alzheimers-dementia/stages

- Washington State has an informative Dementia Advance Directive document to help families plan what is important at all stages of dementia: https://static1.squarespace.com/static/5a0128cf8fd4d22ca11a405d/t/5cd9efd571c10b87c baf4676/1557786582104/dementia-directive.pdf

- Support groups can be a lifesaver. Research has shown that even online resources can be of significant help to caregivers:[15] https://www.alz.org/events/event_search?etid=2&cid=0

- Distinction Between Dementia Symptoms and Alzheimer's Disease Fact Sheet: http://www.dfwsheridan.org/types-dementia or here is a short and sweet definition: Dementia is an overall term used to describe symptoms that impact memory, performance of daily activities, and communication abilities. Alzheimer's disease is the most common type of dementia.

- Helpful 3-minute intro video to Alzheimer's Disease: https://youtu.be/Eq_Er-tqPsA

ABOUT THE CONTRIBUTOR:

Annie Jacobsen is the owner of Jacobsen Dementia Care Coaching www.jacobsendcc.com.

---

[15] https://www.alzheimers.net/internet-based-resources-and-support-for-dementia-caregivers/

CHAPTER 4

ADVANCE CARE PLANNING

onnie Bizzell is memorable. She is high energy, speaks with care and intention, and is great at follow up. I met her at Honoring Choices Pacific Northwest, where she is the Community Engagement Liaison & Program Manager. The Honoring Choices PNW initiative is all about helping people identify what matters most to them, encouraging people to write down their wishes and discuss them with loved ones so that if something happens, decisions might be made in line with wishes.

Advance care planning means thinking about future healthcare decisions that you would want made for you if you couldn't make them yourself. Bonnie said that it is like being prepared for a crisis situation so your loved ones know what is important to you, and they can align decisions to your wishes. Even those working in the healthcare or end-of-life fields, generally don't like to think about, much less plan for an unexpected tragedy.

Bonnie explained that Advance Care Planning is not just documentation, it is a process that includes:

- identifying what is important to you
- describing your wishes of what you want and don't want

- selecting someone you trust to be named as the person to make your healthcare decisions if you are not able to (This person is called a health proxy, health decision surrogate, or power of attorney for healthcare.).

Bonnie shared her personal story, which led her to the work she does today. Her three closest family members each had an unexpected major traumatic medical event – in 2004, 2005 and 2006. Her brother was diagnosed with Crohn's disease and had part of his intestines removed. Her stepdad had a heart attack while he was home alone. He called the ambulance in time to be taken to the hospital and received emergency quadruple bypass surgery. And then her mother had a brain tumor diagnosed, which was a rare form of non-Hodgkin's lymphoma. At the time, only 200 people in the world had been diagnosed with it.

Bonnie's family lived on both coasts of the U.S., and during the three years she cared for her family, she was in and out of three different hospitals. She doesn't remember if anyone in the hospitals asked her family members about advance directives or their wishes. For two of the three family members, there had been no discussion, no thought to what they, as patients, truly wanted. Reflecting on that time, Bonnie shared that if something had happened unexpectedly, she would not have been able to make a decision about what her family members wanted. She did, however, step into the role of patient advocate for those family members, and she learned a lot.

This experience also sparked a desire to make better sense out of the medical system. During the day, Bonnie continued with her project management job in educational assessment, but during her off-hours she began to volunteer at various medical organizations as a family advocate. She used her learning to help make the system more patient-friendly and elevate the voices and needs of other patients. She developed a belief that the way to change healthcare was for patients and families to advocate for themselves. Advance care planning can play a huge role in this by getting people to think, talk, and plan. Bonnie believes advance care planning is not just about how you want to die, but really about how you want to live.

For instance, Bonnie has horrible allergies for which she needs regular medication. She also loves to hike. Sometimes her severe allergies make outdoor activities almost impossible for her to breathe. Knowing that hiking is important, if her doctor offered her a new medication that eliminated her allergy symptoms but had side effects that would prevent her from being able to hike outdoors (like sunlight sensitivity or lethargy), she likely would not choose it.

Medicare will now pay for doctors to have a conversation with patients about end-of-life wishes, if the patient asks for it. But you have to know to ask for that conversation. Too few people actually ever talk about or write down their wishes. As a result, the majority of people do not get the care they want at the end of their life.

WHY IT MATTERS:

- 90% of people say that talking with their loved ones about end-of-life care is important, but only 27% have actually done so, according to The Conversation Project National Survey (2013).[16]

- 82% of people say it's important to put their wishes in writing, but only 23% have actually done so, according to Californians by the California HealthCare Foundation (2012).[17]

- 70% of people say they prefer to die at home, but 60% of people actually die in a long-term care facility or a hospital, according to Californians by the California HealthCare Foundation (2012).[18]

According to the American Hospital Association (2012):[19]

- You are eight times more likely to experience prolonged grief if your loved one dies in the intensive care unit of a hospital, than if he or she died at home with hospice.
- You are five times more likely to experience post-traumatic stress disorder if a loved one dies in an intensive care unit of the hospital than if he or she died at home with hospice.
- Ten fewer days are spent in the hospital during the last two years of life if a patient participated in advance care planning.

USING THIS INFORMATION:

1. Think about advance care planning as a process, not a final decision that you never revisit. Your wishes may change as your life changes.

2. Use family time to talk about your wishes. Don't just leave it to one conversation. You can use the news to solicit your family members' ideas about what is important. Example: "I heard that Aretha Franklin had no will and yet the news reported that they found three wills, each saying something

---

[18] https://www.chcf.org/publication/final-chapter-californians-attitudes-and-experiences-with-death-and-dying/
[19] https://www.aha.org/system/files/2018-02/advanced-illness-management-strategies-2012_0.pdf

different … it made me realize that we all think we know what's going on and sometimes we don't."

3. Not all conversations about wishes need to be serious. For Bonnie and her mom, they regularly discuss what is important and they laugh a lot. She asks her mom about what brings her joy.

4. Think about how your decisions regarding what you do today impact how you want your life to be in the future.

SPECIFIC LANGUAGE YOU CAN USE:

- What brings you joy?
- What three things would you want someone to know about you? What three things *should I* know about you?
- Is there anything you would NOT want, if something unexpected were to happen? (feeding tube, CPR in the hospital, breathing tube, etc.)
- I would like to schedule a doctor visit that includes advanced care planning.

ADDITIONAL READING AND RESOURCES:

- The Hello Game is an interactive tool to help you talk about what matters most (great for families, friends, or communities): https://commonpractice.com/products/hello-game
- The Death Deck is a pack of playing cards that provide a lively game of surprising conversations: https://www.amazon.com/Death-Deck-Lively-Surprising-Conversations/dp/B07GSRDL6H

- *Being Mortal*, is a book by Atul Gawande, who uses compelling storytelling to illustrate how people plan (or don't) at the end of life.
- Honoring Choices website: https://www.honoringchoicespnw.org/
- Five Wishes Advance Directive: https://fivewishes.org/five-wishes/individuals-families/individuals-and-families
- A simple way to document the medical care you would want if you get dementia: https://dementia-directive.org/
- The Final Roadmap is a website that helps families plan and share their wishes, prompted by a series of questions: https://www.finalroadmap.com/

ABOUT THE CONTRIBUTOR:

Bonnie Bizzell, MBA, MEd, is the Community Engagement Liaison & Program Manager for Honoring Choices PNW. www.honoringchoicespnw.org

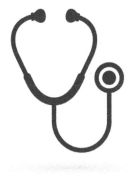

SECTION 2

PARTNERING WITH YOUR DOCTOR

PARTNERING WITH YOUR DOCTOR

Finding a primary care doctor you trust can be challenging, but important. If you have a chronic condition, urgent health issues, or are elderly, a good relationship with your primary care doctor can help you coordinate your care.

If you are not totally honest with your doctor about symptoms or what is happening in your life, you may miss the opportunity to uncover the root of what may be causing illness or disease.

You can interview doctors before becoming a patient. Some doctors will be open to meeting you for a brief introductory visit to see if there is a fit for you in their practice. Remember, doctors can refuse to take you on as a patient!

FOR FURTHER LEARNING:

Schedule for your community or attend The ABCs of an Effective Doctor Visit presentation by a WASHAA representative or speakers available throughout the country: http://www.washaa.org/request-a-presentation.html

ACTION ITEMS:

- ✓ Find and maintain a primary care doctor with whom you can have an honest relationship.

- ✓ Assemble your personal health record, which is all your medical information in one place. This can be paper or electronic. Include information from patient portals, if your health provider uses them. If you are having trouble thinking about the format, WASHAA has a paper copy you can request by contacting info@washaa.org.

- ✓ Make sure that medical information about you is correct. You can often check the accuracy of your information on the patient portal available through your doctor or healthcare system. If there are errors in your records, contact the medical records department to have your records changed.

CHAPTER 5

MISDIAGNOSIS AND LIVING IN THE DIAGNOSIS GREY ZONE

I have known Io Dolka, MS since 2012, when we worked with Beth Droppert, RN, BSN to co-found the Washington State Health Advocacy Association (WASHAA, www.washaa.org). She is recognized as a pioneer in the health advocacy industry and served as the first executive director of WASHAA. Her passion for patient advocacy grew, in part, out of her own experience with a decade-long medical diagnostic odyssey, where she went from bedridden to healthy with the correct diagnosis and treatment. She founded and now runs a Seattle-based medical advocacy company that helps patients navigate missed, inaccurate and delayed diagnosis, and complicated conditions.

Io's company is called GreyZone, because patients who do not fit the black and white criteria used to make a diagnosis often fall in between descriptions and are considered "Grey Zone patients."

Most people don't realize how complicated and difficult arriving at a correct diagnosis can be.[20] As our knowledge of medical conditions is growing every year, available medications

---

[20] https://en.wikipedia.org/wiki/Medical_diagnosis

and treatments are also exponentially improving. Getting it right at the doctor's office is becoming more and more difficult. In fact, 1 out of 20 Americans is misdiagnosed every year.[21]

There are several types of diagnostic error or misdiagnosis:

- **Delayed diagnosis** – when doctors have all the information they need to make a diagnosis but they are delayed in calling it. This can lead to prolonged suffering and further complications from lack of treatment.

- **Missed or incomplete diagnosis** – when providers either completely miss the reason why you are sick or see only part of the reason why a patient experiences their symptoms. Sometimes this happens because diagnostic tests are not accurate or because clinicians are not aware of which tests to run or how to interpret the tests that have been run. An incomplete diagnosis can result in undertreatment or lack of appropriate treatment, and again the chance that more complications will arise from the condition that is going undetected.

- **Wrong diagnosis** – When clinicians assign a wrong diagnosis first before they are able to diagnose the situation accurately. In this circumstance, the mistake can be deadly, like for example when dismissing a sudden and intense headache as a typical migraine rather than a possible stroke, which is an emergency and needs immediate treatment.

Some of the most difficult cases to diagnose are those that deal with the immune system, the endocrine system, or the neurological system, because symptoms can be vague or can change frequently. In those instances, Io said that it is not unusual for people

---

[21] *BMJ Qual Saf* doi:10.1136/bmjqs-2013-002627

to go without a correct diagnosis for 10 years or more. This is also where medical management, the ongoing art of treating diseases and symptoms play a role. According to a recent study from the Mayo Clinic, 88% of all cases that come to the Mayo Clinic for a second opinion receive a revised or different diagnosis, changing the care plan and potentially saving lives.[22]

For women, it is important to realize that most treatments have been tested primarily in men, assuming that how women feel and experience medical conditions may be the same. In 1993, Congress passed a law requiring federally funded research to include women and analyze results by gender, but women are still under represented in research.[23] This also contributes to diagnostic error as providers are not always aware how the same disease can present in men versus women. Heart attacks, are a typical example, where men and women present often with different symptoms.

In chronic, rather than sudden medical situations, diagnosis can be especially difficult. Io shared a story about two of her clients to illustrate how challenging diagnosis can be.

Peggy, a client from New Mexico was in her early twenties … a time in life when people are typically vibrant and healthy. Peggy had longstanding symptoms that included extreme fatigue, anxiety, an inability to concentrate, and frequent difficulty sleeping. Although she had seen several doctors who prescribed antidepressant medicines for her main problem of anxiety, her symptoms were getting progressively worse. Peggy contacted GreyZone after a year and a half of facing these issues because she believed her doctors

[22] https://newsnetwork.mayoclinic.org/discussion/mayo-clinic-researchers-demonstrate-value-of-second-opinions/

[23] https://healthjournalism.org/blog/2018/11/women-more-often-misdiagnosed-because-of-gaps-in-trust-and-knowledge/

were just looking superficially at her symptoms and not trying to find out the root cause of those symptoms.

GreyZone worked with Peggy and her local doctors to order a thorough diagnostic workup that included detailed blood work and to be seen by a team of specialists in the Seattle area. With the additional information garnered from the specialized workup, Peggy was diagnosed with Hashimoto's encephalopathy, a rare autoimmune condition that affects the brain.

With this condition, the body makes antibodies that attack the thyroid and also the brain. Symptoms can include seizures, confusion, or dementia.[24] Interestingly, Peggy's regular thyroid function blood tests were normal, but the blood test for the thyroid antibodies confirmed the diagnosis for this condition. Doctors prescribed specific treatments that were expensive. Peggy wanted to return to her hometown so a local doctor could follow her treatment progress.

Unfortunately, she couldn't find a single doctor in her hometown in New Mexico who was willing to treat her because the treatment was so expensive, the condition was rare, and the treatment was not proven for that condition. Ultimately, she ended up returning to the specialist in Seattle, who put her on the treatment right away. She immediately started getting better. After she completed her treatment, GreyZone identified a doctor back home in New Mexico and GreyZone remained involved remotely to ensure Peggy's needs and priorities were covered while receiving care.

There are other more common conditions that are extremely debilitating but challenging to diagnose because the symptoms come and go or doctors are not aware of the conditions, such as postural orthostatic tachycardia syndrome (POTS) which causes a rapidly accelerating heartbeat. According to Dysautonomia International, POTS is estimated to affect 1 out of 100 teenagers and, including

---

[24] https://www.verywellhealth.com/hashimotos-encephalopathy-overview-3231700

adult patients, a total of 1 million to 3 million Americans. It is most frequently seen in young women, often less than 35 years of age.

Olivia, another client of Io's, in her mid-30s, first experienced what felt like panic attacks out of the blue, with a racing heart and the feeling of not being able to catch her breath. Olivia couldn't work because of this condition, so it was very impactful on her life. She couldn't take care of her family, and financially things were very difficult. Initial consultations with general practitioners claimed it was due to anxiety and they treated her with antidepressants. But Olivia's symptoms grew worse, including extreme fatigue and difficulty walking long distances. Doctors then believed her symptoms were most likely caused by depression and there also might be an issue with her heart, so they sent her to a cardiologist who did some basic testing to rule out arrhythmia, which is an abnormal heart rhythm. But the doctor said, according to the tests, everything was okay.

With her previous diagnostic tests in hand, Olivia contacted GreyZone looking for help in getting the right diagnosis. Io's team at GreyZone reviewed her history and diagnostic information and immediately saw red flags. They asked Olivia to keep track of her heart rate and record when she felt her heart racing. It seemed that every time Olivia was out walking, she would feel a panic attack, and her heart would race. A normal person's heart rate is about 80 beats per minute. Every time Olivia would arise from a chair, her heart would beat about 130 or 140 beats per minute. She was dizzy and exhausted.

With her new information in hand, GreyZone sent Olivia to a subspecialist in cardiology for further specialized testing, which could pinpoint the correct diagnosis: POTS. It took a few months to figure out the best treatments. Doctors prescribed medications and she changed her lifestyle which dramatically improved her quality of life. She gradually regained her stamina, her ability to stand for longer periods of time, and was able to reduce her heart rate. Those improvements allowed her to resume a normal life after a few months.

Io suggests the following actions to help you advocate well for yourself when seeking the right diagnosis:

1. Seek a second opinion for long-term symptoms without diagnosis or with diagnosis and no improvement.
2. Seek immediate help if your condition deteriorates quickly.
3. Find an advocate who can help you navigate the maze if you feel overwhelmed.
4. Know thyself! Monitor symptoms, cause and effect, keep diaries, describe your symptoms with detail and clarity, and provide as much information to the doctors as possible.
5. Keep at it. Connect with online or face-to-face communities for support.
6. Take care of yourself if you have a GreyZone condition as it usually takes its toll emotionally, physically and financially.
7. Your family or support system needs to get support as well. Your condition impacts those around you.

WHY IT MATTERS:

- Diagnostic errors may be more harmful to patients than treatment mistakes. A Johns Hopkins study reported 80,000 to 160,000 patients suffer misdiagnosis-related, potentially preventable, significant permanent injury or death annually in the United States. [25]

---

[25] https://www.hopkinsmedicine.org/news/media/releases/diagnostic_errors_more_common_costly_and_harmful_than_treatment_mistakes

- The Institute of Medicine estimates that more than half the US population will suffer from at least one wrong or delayed diagnosis during their lifetime.

- Most people are not aware of how difficult it is to make a correct diagnosis. It is not typically simple, and the majority of medicine actually functions within the GreyZone, according to Amitabh Chandra, PhD, professor of public policy at Harvard Kennedy School.[26]

USING THIS INFORMATION:

1. Consider a second opinion for any major medical diagnosis. In a study from the Mayo Clinic, only 12 percent of patients seeking a second opinion were correctly diagnosed by their primary care doctor. Surprisingly, 21% percent (one in five people in the study) were misdiagnosed, leading to higher costs, too.[27]

2. Sudden, severe, worsening symptoms (such as sharp pain or not being able to walk) should be seen immediately by a medical professional. If you aren't able to reach your doctor, go to the emergency room.

3. Io recommends that patients always gather all documents related to their medical records. Because it can be thousands of pages for complicated patients, it is good to organize your records. Hire an advocate to do that if you are not able to do it yourself. That will help every doctor to actually read them.

---

[26] https://www.medscape.com/viewarticle/844348
[27] https://onlinelibrary.wiley.com/doi/full/10.1111/jep.12747

4. Sometimes it is hard to be accepted into the Mayo Clinic and other institutions that take on difficult cases. Seek consultations at academic institutions locally instead, or ask your insurance provider for second opinion benefits.

SPECIFIC LANGUAGE YOU CAN USE:

- What else could this be?
- Could two things be going on at the same time?
- Are there other tests or significant false positives/negatives in my current tests that should be initiated or redone (maybe by another lab)?
- Are the images taken good and clear? How can I explore securing a second person to read them?
- Before I choose treatment, what other options do I have that we have not explored?
- Thank you for your opinion. I value it and because our next step is so serious and important, I would like to get a second opinion. I would like to get copies of my tests. Are there other things I should look at to get a full picture of my options?

ADDITIONAL READING AND RESOURCES:

- This "Checklist for Getting the Right Diagnosis" adapted from the National Patient Safety Foundation and the Society to Improve Diagnosis in Medicine: http://www.nationalacademies.org/hmd/Reports/2015/Improving-Diagnosis-in-Healthcare/~/media/BAD554B1BB1546D38C9BC281D6671775.ashx

- "Should I Ask for a Second Opinion?" https://www.aarp. org/health/conditions-treatments/info-2017/second-diagnosis-saves-lives-fd.html
- WASHAA 2nd opinion webinar http://www.washaa.org/ ceus-second-opinion.html
- Resource for Patients – Society to Improve Diagnosis in Medicine https://www.improvediagnosis.org/patientresources/

ABOUT THE CONTRIBUTOR:

Io Dolka is the Founder and Chief Care Advocate of GreyZone, LLC. Patient stories are used with her permission. More information is available at www.GreyZoneHealth.com.

CHAPTER 6

OVERDIAGNOSIS: WHEN A DIAGNOSIS MIGHT NOT REQUIRE TREATMENT

David Ansley had been a healthcare editor and reporter for decades when I met him in 2017 through his work at *Consumer Reports* and the Choosing Wisely campaign. The campaign has excellent, easy-to-understand materials and advice on how to ask questions about whether care or treatment is really needed. I was interested to hear about David's personal experience with this issue.

In September of 2002, after returning from a Labor Day weekend hiking trip in the mountains, David woke up with a numb left hand and painful left elbow, rendering that arm useless. Since David was a writer and couldn't use his hand, much less type, he had to call in sick. He took a sick day, thinking he could rest his arm to recover quickly and wondered what he might have done to cause such a severe symptom.

After a day or two of rest and aspirin, the pain seemed to be worsening. He went to his usual clinic, but his regular doctor was on vacation, so he saw a new doctor. She took his symptoms seriously. She did a thorough neurological work-up and explained her hunch; it had something to do with the arm nerves emerging from the upper spine. She ordered an MRI, and luckily there was a portable MRI unit in a big trailer parked behind the office building that day. They could see him immediately.

It was the first time David had experienced an MRI, and as he went through the procedure, he said he felt very powerless and unbelieving that something could be seriously wrong. Yet, he couldn't figure out what he might have done to cause the pain. When the MRI was complete, the technician said that a radiologist read the scan immediately and had seen something puzzling. He now wanted to capture an image of the lower spine with contrast agent. The technician asked if David was okay with proceeding? There was no doctor available to discuss this decision to proceed or not. No one had accompanied David to this appointment, since he hadn't thought it would be a big deal. He felt he had to decide on the spot.

He decided to proceed. After the second procedure, the technician said that the radiologist would read the image and call David's doctor. David went home feeling puzzled and concerned.

The next day, the doctor who had examined him called him at home and asked David to "sit down." She said that he had a diagnosis of something she had never seen before and that he should not look it up on the Internet. She said he had a syrinx in his lower back. The doctor said that she had made a referral to a neurologist for an appointment in eight to 10 days and that the neurologist would take it from there. David asked why this syrinx would impact his arm, hand and elbow, since that made little sense physiologically. David said that he felt like she was washing her hands of the situation, because she didn't have an answer and wouldn't speculate.

In the meantime, David did look up syrinx on the Internet, and what he read was "really scary."

He learned that a syrinx is a fluid-filled gap down the middle of the spinal cord. It can be present from birth or caused later by an injury or a tumor. While the early symptoms may be weakness and insensitivity to pain, the condition typically worsens. Pressure on the nerves causes muscle spasms and unrelenting pain. There's no real cure, and some people with a syrinx end their own lives.

Because of his line of work, David knows a lot of doctors. With more than a week before his appointment with the neurologist and feeling terrified, he called a doctor friend in New York. She didn't mock the diagnosis, but she wondered aloud if the pain could instead be caused by inflammation somewhere else. She asked David if he would try Motrin to see if that would help. He did so, and the pain seemed to get a little better.

At his neurology appointment, the neurologist asked David to repeat his story about his pain and what had been happening right before he experienced the pain's onset. The doctor manipulated the elbow and tapped David's knees. He then displayed the MRI image and showed David where in his spine the syrinx was located. Because of the sudden onset and location of the pain, he said, the syrinx was likely something David had from birth – unrelated to the arm pain, causing no symptoms, and at this point unlikely to cause any harm at all.

The doctor asked David if he had experienced his left shoulder tightly compressing before the pain started. David suddenly remembered that the backpack he was using during the hiking trip was borrowed from someone else and hadn't fit well. His shoulder had felt pinched. The neurologist said that in fact, he thought David had a pinched nerve and he would be fine in a week or so. This is exactly what happened.

In asking David how he might have reacted to this scenario knowing what he does now, he responded by saying:

- "Just because you find something, don't assume that it is bad. There are many tests that find things like slow-growing cancers or birth defects, that had they never been found, might never have created symptoms.

- A syrinx was such a rare condition that, at the time, the only information was on poor outcomes, not the whole range of experience. Today, online descriptions acknowledge that a syrinx can be discovered on unrelated MRI scans and, if not causing problems, can just be monitored.

- If something doesn't make sense or isn't logical, listen to yourself and push to understand what is happening with your body."

The National Institutes of Health defines overdiagnosis as the diagnosis of a medical condition that would never have caused any symptoms or problems. This kind of diagnosis can be harmful if it leads to psychological stress and unnecessary treatments.

It's important to know that overdiagnosis is not the same as misdiagnosis. Misdiagnosis is a wrong diagnosis. For instance, if someone is diagnosed with cancer but they have a benign cyst. Overdiagnosis is a "correct" medical diagnosis.

WHY IT MATTERS:

Although difficult to quantify, overdiagnosis occurs when a true abnormality is discovered, but detection of that abnormality does not benefit the patient. It should be distinguished from misdiagnosis, in which the diagnosis is inaccurate, and it is not the same as overtreatment or overuse, in which excess medication or procedures are provided to patients for both correct and incorrect diagnoses.

Overdiagnosis for adult conditions has gained a great deal of recognition over the last few years, led by realizations that certain screening initiatives, such as those for breast and prostate cancer, may be harming the very people they were designed to protect.

There are certain conditions where overdiagnosis is rampant:

- ADHD[28]
- breast cancer[29]
- prostate cancer[30]
- thyroid cancer[31]

USING THIS INFORMATION:

Carefully considering the benefits and drawbacks of screening tests can help you reach the best decision for you:

1. Would you rather have regular screening tests, even if that means risking overdiagnosis, with all the physical and psychological consequences?

2. Or would you prefer to avoid unnecessary diagnoses and treatments, even if that means that a serious illness might only be discovered at a later stage, when treatment may be less effective?

---

[28] https://www.health.harvard.edu/blog/is-adhd-overdiagnosed-and-overtreated-2017031611304

[29] http://tcr.amegroups.com/article/view/24419/html

[30] https://www.sciencedaily.com/releases/2017/01/170109190333.htm

[31] https://journals.plos.org/plosone/article?id=10.1371/journal.pone.0179387

SPECIFIC LANGUAGE YOU CAN USE:

- How do you compare treatment and non-treatment with my overall projected life expectancy?
- How will this treatment's likely side effects compare with not receiving treatment?
- If I had not known about this diagnosis, how soon would it likely have been before I would notice symptoms, and what would they be?
- What would happen if I wait? What are the next steps?
- If I wait until another stage of progression, what are my chances that the treatment would be more or less effective?

ADDITIONAL READING AND RESOURCES:

- "Overdiagnosis, What It Is and What It Isn't" https://ebm.bmj.com/content/23/1/1
- "How Much Are We Over-Diagnosing Cancer?" https://www.forbes.com/sites/peterubel/2015/05/22/the-question-isnt-whether-we-are-overdiagnosing-cancer-but-how-much/#7cbaf8b579b0
- "ADHD is Now Widely Overdiagnosed and For Multiple Reasons" https://www.psychologytoday.com/us/blog/side-effects/201710/adhd-is-now-widely-overdiagnosed-and-multiple-reasons
- *Improving quality by doing less: overdiagnosis.* Ebell M, Herzstein J, Am Fam Physician. 2015 Feb 1; 91(3):162-3.

ABOUT THE CONTRIBUTOR:

David Ansley is a healthcare editor and reporter and can be reached at: ansley.david@gmail.com. His story is used with permission.

CHAPTER 7

OVERTREATMENT:
IS THIS MEDICINE NECESSARY?

Gene, a former boxer, and my athletic trainer, grew up England. He was a world-ranked professional boxer, who trained in Seattle, Atlanta, Dallas, Philadelphia, New York and LA. Because we have been training together for years, we talk about all kinds of things: politics, movies and health. He also loves to compare England to America.

In his early 40s, Gene was the picture of health standing at over six feet tall. However, he had a hidden health problem that men generally don't like to discuss, now solved due to his diligence in trying to find an answer.

Gene's problem of needing to use the bathroom almost hourly really affected his life, especially waking up several times in the middle of the night. Typically, this is a sign of serious trouble with the prostate. Gene went to three different doctors for a diagnosis and suffered the indignities that most people do while trying to find out what was wrong. Gene said the urine and bladder tests by doctors led to a diagnosis of overactive bladder. They told Gene he was eliminating similarly to a 70-year old man. Each of the doctors gave Gene medicines to try to solve the problem. He didn't know to ask if his symptoms could mean a different diagnosis.

Gene didn't want to take bladder medicine as he was already taking allergy medicine and felt strongly that he wanted to find an alternative to taking additional medicine. He observed, "Americans use 47% of all pharmaceuticals in the world, and now I know why." As Gene said, "I didn't want to be taking loads of medicines at my age if I didn't have to."

Gene did some research and found that heavyweight boxers who have compromised their abdominal wall because of intense abdominal training can destroy bladder muscles. He found that doing Kegel exercises might help. Kegel exercises are simple clench-and-release exercises that you can do to make the muscles of your pelvic floor stronger. [32] "To start, I couldn't even do one Kegel exercise ... but after a while I got better." Without the pills and with the exercises, Gene reported that he slept through the night and this impactful issue was no longer a problem.

WHY IT MATTERS:

- Americans are taking more prescription pills than ever before — and taking more than people in any other country. *Consumer Reports* warns that all those pills may not be necessary and might do more harm than good.[33]

- The number of prescriptions filled by Americans each year, for both adults and children, has soared by 85 percent over two decades — from 2.4 billion in 1997 to 4.5 billion in 2016, according to the heath research firm Quintile IMS.

---

[32] https://www.healthline.com/health/kegel-exercises
[33] https://www.consumerreports.org/media-room/press releases/2017/08/consumer_reports_examines_do_americans_take_too_many_prescription_medications/

Meanwhile, the US population increased by only 21 percent during that time. Much of that medication is lifesaving or at least life-improving. But many medications are not necessary or effective.

USING THIS INFORMATION:

1. *Consumer Reports* identifies 12 situations in which people can try lifestyle changes to address symptoms rather than risking the possible side effects of medication; they include:

   - ADHD
   - back and joint pain
   - dementia
   - mild depression
   - heartburn
   - insomnia
   - low testosterone
   - osteopenia
   - overactive bladder
   - prediabetes
   - prehypertension
   - obesity[34]

2. Don't cut back or stop taking a drug without first discussing it with your doctor.

3. Have a comprehensive drug review with your doctor or pharmacist at least once a year.

---

[34] https://www.consumerreports.org/prescription-drugs/times-to-try-lifestyle-changes-before-drugs/

SPECIFIC LANGUAGE YOU CAN USE:

- Are there any other options (like lifestyle changes) other than this prescribed drug that will help my situation?
- What if I don't take this drug?
- Is it possible to decrease this or other drugs?

ADDITIONAL READING AND RESOURCES:

- "How to Get Off Prescription Drugs" https://www.consumer reports.org/prescription-drugs/how-to-get-off-prescription -drugs/
- "Give Your Drugs a Checkup: Reviewing Your Medicine List Can Prevent Errors" https://www.consumerreports.org/prescription-drugs/reviewing-your-medication-list-can-prevent-errors/
- "Stop Taking Too Many Medicines" https://www.people spharmacy.com/2017/10/30/is-a-loved-one-taking-too -many-medicines/
- "How Many Pills are Too Many?" https://www.nytimes.com/2017/04/10/upshot/how-many-pills-are-too-many.html?_r=0

CHAPTER 8

WHEN TO FIRE THE DOCTOR

My good friend, Rabbi Allison Flash, and her family have had more than their share of medical challenges. She has had lots of experience with doctors and hospitals, and she shared with me a story from her early years as a mother when she was new to navigating healthcare.

In 2007, her youngest son Daniel was just three years old when their family of five moved from Nashville, Tennessee to Seattle. Very shortly after the move, Daniel spiked a fever that wouldn't go away. Allison took Daniel to the pediatrician who referred them to the children's hospital in Seattle. Although he had no respiratory symptoms, after a battery of tests, it turned out that eighty percent of Daniel's lungs were infiltrated with something, they just didn't know what.

At 7:00 p.m. that night, the hospital pulmonologist called Allison at home and said it was urgent to bring Daniel to the hospital right away. They would be observing Daniel and then run tests early the next morning. Allison's husband was traveling, so after arranging for Daniel's siblings to stay with Allison's sister-in-law, they were off to the hospital. Allison said that she felt very alone in the hospital with her son, having just moved to town, waiting and worrying, while her husband tried to figure out the next flight home from Florida.

Allison had been up all night, so when the pulmonologist walked into Daniel's hospital room the next morning and said he was sure Daniel had Wegener's disease, which is terminal (meaning her son would die from this disease), she didn't know what hit her. In addition to this horrible news, it was *how* the news was delivered that especially angered her. Allison said that the pulmonologist didn't sit down. He didn't ask if she had questions. He didn't explain the disease in detail. He just walked in, stood at the bedside looking down at them and said he was sorry her son had a terminal disease and then left. It stunned her. (Note: Wegener's Disease is an uncommon inflammatory disease, and people who have it are at high risk of dying within two years.)[35]

As the day went on, different specialists from different departments in the hospital came to see Daniel, and every one of them stated that they were sure it was something other than Wegener's Disease; they just didn't know what. Some of these specialists were Chairs of their departments. However, the pulmonologist insisted that this diagnosis was correct, and he was the leader in their case. The pulmonologist did not come to see Allison or Daniel again, so they couldn't ask questions. Allison didn't know what to do.

Fortunately, Allison's father is a retired physician and she called him. In all of his years in practice, he had never seen a case of Wegener's. Her father also consulted his best friend who was a retired pediatric physician. He too had never seen a case of Wegener's because it was so rare. However, the pulmonologist had dug in his heels on the diagnosis. Allison reflected that, "it felt like he was writing a paper on Wegener's and needed a subject – forcing

---

our child to have something he didn't have. He was so abrupt about it, and he was so sure of himself, but it made me wonder."

What was most striking to Allison was that the doctor never sat down, and he never listened. He never gave her the sense he was hearing what she wanted to know. Although the other doctors were extra kind and didn't come out and say the pulmonologist was wrong, they also assured Allison that they did not believe it was Wegener's.

Allison said that if she hadn't previously had experience advocating for her children in a medical setting, knowing to trust her gut, or if she didn't know that it was okay to speak up and ask questions, she would have been convinced that her child was dying.

Allison felt like she wasn't complaining but asked questions of the specialists about the pulmonologist's diagnosis and manner. She said that the specialists gave a knowing look and while they did not criticize the doctor, it felt like they were going out of their way to make it up to Allison's family for the other doctor allowing the family to believe that Daniel had a terminal disease.

The next day, Daniel had to undergo an invasive test that required him to be sedated under general anesthesia. Fortunately for the family, the original pulmonologist was not available to do the procedure and a different pulmonologist stepped in.

Allison's husband had made it back to Seattle, and he and Allison were in the waiting room anxious to hear about how Daniel's procedure went. The new doctor entered, sat with them and spoke plain English. He explained what had been done and what the medical staff were going to need to do next. He assured Allison and her husband that their son did not have Wegener's.

At that point Allison looked at the doctor and asked if he would take the case over from the previous pulmonologist. She also calmly requested that the first doctor never, ever touch Daniel again.

What Allison learned from that experience was that if the doctor isn't treating you with respect, refuses to listen to you, or makes you feel like you have no voice in the conversation, it is time to get a new doctor.

In the end, there never was a definitive diagnosis for Allison's son. Although, the second pulmonologist, who happened to be from the Nashville area, thought it likely was a fungus that is common to that area. In the end, the original pulmonologist transferred to another hospital out of town and focused on research instead of treating patients.

WHY IT MATTERS:

- Trust between doctors and patients is important to getting the best care possible. Yet, almost a quarter (23%) of Americans are not always truthful with their doctors , according to a 2019 study conducted by TermLife2Go.[36] This can lead to mis-, over-, or delayed diagnosis, or treatment options that might not be optimal.

- Your ability to communicate effectively with your doctor can affect your care. The three main goals of doctor-patient communication are: creating a good interpersonal relationship, facilitating exchange of information, and including patients in decision making. A patient's agreement with the doctor about the nature of the treatment and the need for follow-up is strongly associated with their recovery.[37]

USING THIS INFORMATION:

There are few relationships as intimate and important as your relationship with your doctor. The example above shows why trust in

---

[36] termlife2go.com/lying-to-your-doctor
[37] https://www.ncbi.nlm.nih.gov/pmc/articles/PMC3096184/

your doctor, good communication, and alignment of your values are important. Here are some instances when you might want to consider changing doctors:

1. **Your doctor doesn't listen to your concerns.** If you feel rushed, or the doctor shuts you down when you ask questions, this relationship might not be a good fit. Find out if it is just a particular day or situation, or if this is the norm for the doctor. You can ask for more time or ask if the doctor will allow you to put forth all your questions. If the doctor doesn't have a good answer, look for another doctor.

2. **Your doctor doesn't use plain language you can understand**. If your doctor is using words or language that is confusing to you, ask the doctor to write down the diagnosis and explain it to you in plain language. If the doctor is struggling to explain it, ask him or her to draw a picture or explain it to you as if you are the doctor's grandmother. Sometimes two people don't communicate well for a variety of reasons. If this happens, you can let the doctor know that you are not understanding, and it is important to you to understand things before you make a medical decision. You can also bring someone along to help prompt the doctor to explain something in another way.

3. **You feel the doctor's behavior is disrespectful**. Standing over you, not listening, yelling at you or their staff could be signs that the doctor may be struggling. Stay calm and speak with either the head nurse or attending physician at the hospital to request another doctor take your case. This is also true for nurses who are disrespectful. You can request that a nurse not work with you. As the patient or family member, remember to be calm, direct, and compassionate,

as well. If you have multiple requests to not work with staff, those requests may not necessarily be granted. If this is the case, you may want to examine your own contribution to the situation.

SPECIFIC LANGUAGE YOU CAN USE:

To help you clarify what the doctor is telling you, here are some ways to phrase your questions:

- Can you help me understand what the goal of the treatment is?
- Can you tell me in plain language what this diagnosis means?
- Could this possibly be something else?

If a doctor is not treating you with the respect you feel you deserve, be direct and calmly state:

- I would like you to understand this from my perspective. I feel confused/angry/sad and would like to (state an action such as: pause, regroup, learn more, seek a second opinion, have another specialist's point of view) in order to (state your goal such as: live my life without feeling sick, extend my life, understand my options and next steps).
- The way you stated things upset me, because although you might deliver this news all day to patients, this is a first-time experience for me. I would like to have more time and your direct attention so I can ask questions

and know that you are hearing what I am saying (or asking). Does that make sense? Is this something you can do with me?

- I have a lot to think about, and I would like to talk through with you how your recommendations/observations/diagnosis fit with my goals/values/hopes. Can you help me do that? If not, is there someone else who can?

For your regular doctor, there is no need to get into a discussion if you are convinced you need to change to a new doctor, but you will want to make sure you have found another doctor first. Then, ask your regular doctor's office to transfer your medical records. They have an obligation to do this.

ADDITIONAL READING AND RESOURCES:

- "How to Fire Your Doctor. Rule One: Make Sure You Have Another One Lined Up First" https://www.washingtonpost.com/national/health-science/how-to-fire-your-doctor-rule-one-make-sure-you-have-another-one-lined-up-first/2014/01/13/44778c2e-76fb-11e3-af7f-13bf0e9965f6_story.html?noredirect=on&utm_term=.e645c3cf8316

- "Giving Your Doctor the Pink Slip" Center for Advancing Health http://www.cfah.org/prepared-patient/prepared-patient-articles/giving-your-doctor-the-pink-slip

- "12 Signs You Should Fire Your Doctor" https://health.usnews.com/health-care/patient-advice/slideshows/signs-you-should-fire-your-doctor?onepage

- "9 Signs You Should Fire Your Doctor" https://www.nextavenue.org/fire-your-doctor/

- "Women are more likely than men to lie to doctors" https://www.zocdoc.com/about/news/new-zocdoc-study-reveals-women-are-more-likely-than-men-to-lie-to-doctors/

- "When Evidence Says No, but Doctors Say Yes" https://www.theatlantic.com/health/archive/2017/02/when-evidence-says-no-but-doctors-say-yes/517368/

- "Reasons for Switching Doctors" https://www.verywell-health.com/is-it-time-to-change-doctors-2615476

- "13 Reasons Why Patients Change Doctors" (from 1957 and just for fun) https://www.ncbi.nlm.nih.gov/pmc/articles/PMC2641051/pdf/jnma00715-0038.pdf

ABOUT THE CONTRIBUTOR:

Rabbi Allison Flash has given permission to cite her son's story.

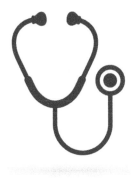

SECTION 3

BEING PREPARED IN THE HOSPITAL

BEING PREPARED IN THE HOSPITAL

In 2009 I was attending the National Association of Healthcare Advocacy (NAHAC) second annual meeting, and there I listened intently to speaker Karen Curtiss who was sharing her story. She had multiple family members who had been hospitalized. Some survived and some did not. In memory of those who had experienced close calls and her father Bill Aydt, who died, she founded the nonprofit organization CampaignZERO. There were several elements to her presentation which lit a fire inside of me:

- Death from preventable medical errors in the hospital is the third leading cause of death in the United States, right behind heart disease and cancer.[38]

- The death rate is equivalent to three Boeing 747 airplanes crashing every day with no survivors.

- She shared two versions of a patient story, called "Sarah's Story." One version unfolding as it normally would, with the

---

[38] Makary MA, Daniel M. BMJ. 2016 May 3, 353: i2139. doi: 10.1136/bmj.i2139.

patient's care partner not knowing how to help. The second version of the story showed how practical tips learned through CampaignZero checklists could help avoid certain known hazards in the hospital.

The CampaignZero presentation, Safe & Sound in the Hospital: A Short Course in Patient Safety, is still one of my favorite presentations because it is very empowering to people. It is chock-full of helpful tips and checklists.

By reading this section, you will learn a few of the top concerns in the hospital. Believe me, there are many more, but I hope that by reading these chapters you will become more observant, more involved, and develop confidence in asking questions.

FOR FURTHER LEARNING:

✓ Attend Safe & Sound in the Hospital: A Short Course in Patient Safety. You can find a list of community educators here: https://www.campaignzero.org/our-community-educators/

✓ CampaignZero.org has several checklists.

ACTION ITEMS:

✓ Always have on hand a Hospital Ready Bag, should you have to go to the hospital unexpectedly. I recommend that you include in this bag:

- THIS BOOK!
- your personal health record, including your list of medications and any over the counter (drugstore) medications you've taken in the past three months: things like nicotine patches, headache, cold and sinus remedies, minerals and vitamins.

- copies of CampaignZERO's hospital safety checklists (free!), downloadable at CampaignZERO.org.
- wipes and spray cleaners (both bleach and anti-bacterial). See CampaignZERO's checklists about preventing infection!
- a big bottle of antimicrobial hand cleanser (like Purell)
- socks with non-skid rubber on the bottom

CHAPTER 9

CODE STATUS: DETERMINING YOUR CODE STATUS IN THE HOSPITAL

In this chapter, we discuss what code status is and why it is vitally important that you know about it before you go to the hospital. Dr. Charles Pilcher is a retired emergency room physician and Hospital Board Member of Evergreen Health. He chairs the hospital's Board Quality Committee, consults on medical malpractice and is passionate about educating the public about what happens in the hospital if they code.

First, it is important to understand what code means: it means your heart stops beating. Most of us would not think about the possibility of that happening, until we are admitted into the hospital. There, they will ask what you want to happen if your heart stops – or you "code". Do you want CPR? Dr. Pilcher says that most people, if offered CPR in that instance, believe that this a good choice. However, most people don't have a clear picture of what being "coded" means – and if they did, they might reconsider. For some people, being admitted to the hospital is the first time they may have had to consider this potential scenario.

Some common side effects of CPR include broken ribs or lung puncture, especially in older patients with frail bones.

Dr. Pilcher says that even if ribs are not broken, a very sore chest is a certainty.

Admitting forms typically ask patients if they want:

- No Code: Nothing will be done to artificially restart your heart. This is also called "Do Not Resuscitate," or "DNR."
- Modified Code: Do Not Intubate, or Do Not do CPR or some version of this.
- Full Code: Everything will be done to try to restart your heart.

In a full code situation, Dr. Pilcher explains that patients typically believe "Full Code" is a good option, the presumption being that this intervention will be successful. However, the reality is that the statistics are grim. Ninety percent of all people who code don't survive. Because of this, most hospitals have instituted Rapid Response Teams to evaluate and treat patients when they first begin to show signs that they are getting worse. The goal is to prevent the "code" in the first place.

Here are two patient stories from Dr. Pilcher:

Gladys, a mother in her late 70s with ovarian cancer and lung metastases, was admitted into the hospital for trouble breathing. When presented with the code form and asked about her "Code Status," Gladys thought "Of course I want to be resuscitated! Why else would I be here in the hospital?" Gladys elected to be "Full Code."

Gladys had three daughters, two of whom lived in town and were close to her. Her third daughter lived out of town, and they were not close emotionally.

Two days after Gladys was admitted to the hospital, she experienced cardiac arrest and because she chose Full Code, the cardiac arrest code team started doing CPR. They successfully restarted her heart, but she did not resume breathing on her own, so she was intubated (a tube was inserted) and put on a ventilator. Gladys remained unconscious in the hospital bed with her two daughters bedside her. The third daughter said she would fly in, and "Whatever you do, don't take Mom off the ventilator until I arrive."

Gladys was in the hospital's the Intensive Care Unit (ICU), heavily sedated, her blood pressure and vital signs were unstable, and she had broken ribs from the CPR. Gladys was experiencing extreme pain. The third daughter arrived two days later and wanted Gladys to wake up so she could say goodbye and make amends because she hadn't seen Gladys in a few years. But Gladys remained on a ventilator and couldn't speak. The sisters disagreed about taking Gladys off the ventilator.

When Gladys went into cardiac arrest again five days later, she could not be resuscitated. Gladys died having spent an extra week in the hospital in extreme pain. Had her family understood that the likelihood of success for CPR is only 10%, might they have chosen a different treatment plan?

Contrast that with another patient, a 90-year old woman named Molly who had late stage Alzheimer's disease and lived in a nursing home. Molly came to the emergency room running a fever, and a chest X-ray confirmed she had pneumonia. Molly's life in the nursing home was limited to lying in a fetal position, unaware of her surroundings. Since Molly's family was not with her, the emergency physician's quandary was: Do I assume Molly wants to die a natural death, i.e., death from pneumonia, or do I treat the pneumonia? Fortunately, Molly's son arrived before the doctor had to make that decision. The son and the doctor had a conversation, and the son agreed that Molly had a terrible quality of life in the nursing home and would prefer to die naturally. Molly's pneumonia was not treated, and she died a natural death less than 24 hours later.

Dr. Pilcher described to me what happens when someone's heart stops:

When a patient's heart stops, the hospital will alert staff to a code by pager, overhead speakers, or other technology to signify that someone's heart has stopped. About a half dozen staff respond, and one will push on the chest about one hundred times a minute. A tube is inserted through the mouth and into the lungs to provide oxygen. Sometimes the defibrillator is necessary if the heart is fibrillating (having a rapid, non-functional rhythm). A current of electricity is passed through the chest and heart, which may or may not restart normal heart activity. Sometimes there are un-shockable heart rhythms that respond better to CPR or drugs. The heart may resume beating – or it may not. The patient may resume breathing – or they may not. The second possibility is by far more likely.

WHY IT MATTERS:

- Patients may not understand the risks of CPR in the hospital. According to one study, patients estimated their own likelihood of survival after CPR would be 70%, while the real survival if CPR is administered in the hospital is about 10 – 15%.[39] Interestingly, CPR performed outside the hospital may have a higher likelihood of survival. [40]

- Medical residents who discuss these decisions with patients inform them of potential outcomes of their code decisions less than one-third of the time, according to a study.[41]

---

[39] https://www.ncbi.nlm.nih.gov/pubmed/9686710?dopt=Abstract
[40] According to 2014 data, nearly 45 percent of out-of-hospital cardiac arrest victims survived when bystander CPR was administered (American Heart Association)
[41] https://www.ncbi.nlm.nih.gov/pmc/articles/PMC4000342/

USING THIS INFORMATION:

1. Understanding what you want in terms of resuscitation in the hospital is important. Dr. Pilcher suggests that if you are on a downward trajectory with increasingly diminished quality of life (e.g., end stage renal disease, end state congestive heart failure, COPD, end stage cancer), you should consider choosing a natural death rather than all measures to restart your heart. Once you make that decision, opting for maximum comfort through palliative care (comfort care) or home hospice is an excellent option.

2. You should ask your health care provider to complete a Physician's Order for Life-Sustaining Treatment (POLST, as it is called in Washington), available in most states. This is done in your physician's office and supersedes a living will or previous DNR form. The form is lime green, requires a physician to fill it out and sign it, and is generally used by older people who do not want to be resuscitated if something happens. People generally post this on their refrigerator door, so it is easily found by paramedics. Discuss this option with your healthcare provider.

3. If you are a young, generally healthy person who is, for example, going into the hospital for a knee replacement, Dr. Pilcher says that choosing to be "Full Code" is perfectly appropriate.

4. If you or your loved one is in the hospital and unsure of your chances of meaningful survival or what your code status should be, ask more questions. First ask your nurse, then your doctor, then the charge nurse, then the nursing supervisor. If you still have questions, ask for a second opinion. Making decisions should be easy. It's getting the information you need that's hard.

SPECIFIC LANGUAGE YOU CAN USE:

- What does my code status selection mean?
- What will it mean if I need to be on a ventilator? Will I be able to talk?
- Do you have a rapid response team here? How does it work?
- How do I know if I am at risk of a cardiac arrest?
- Can you have my doctor come in and talk with me about the plan of care?

ADDITIONAL READING AND RESOURCES:

- Additional cases illustrating do not resuscitate and CPR perceptions of doctors and patients from Agency for Healthcare Research and Quality: https://psnet.ahrq.gov/webmm/case/25/code-status-confusion
- *Knocking on Heaven's Door*, by Katy Butler: https://www.goodreads.com/en/book/show/16130658-knocking-on-heaven-s-door

ABOUT THE CONTRIBUTOR:

Charles Pilcher MD FACEP is a retired emergency room physician, ER medical director, and Emergency Medical Malpractice Expert Witness.

CHAPTER 10

CLEAN SURFACES: YOU CAN HELP PREVENT INFECTION

Linda Lybert is an expert in health surface materials and how to keep surfaces clean. She has had a fascinating career that led to founding the Health Surfaces Institute, whose mission is: to reduce preventable infections through a collaboration of industry, academia, science, regulatory, and service sectors by interrupting the transmission of surface-related pathogens in healthcare to support community health. She shared with me very valuable information and advice about the role patients and family members can play in preventing infection, especially in the hospital.

Linda started our conversation by stating that most people do not realize that hospital acquired- infections (HAIs) are the fourth leading cause of death in the United States and that surfaces are the foundational issue. Surfaces in the healthcare environment are contaminated, and because we cannot see microbes, they are difficult if not impossible to clean, let alone disinfect. She explained that infection-causing microbes are transferred from surfaces to hands, and then to the patient.

Linda and a colleague were shopping and talking about her work. While in the store, a young woman in her 30s approached Linda with tears in her eyes and simply said, "Thank you." Linda wondered aloud to the woman what she should be thanked for? The woman said that she and her fiancé were in the final stages of planning their upcoming wedding when he went into the hospital for a simple outpatient surgery. He was dead three days later because of an infection he got while in surgery. In thanking Linda, the young woman was grateful that someone was working to make sure patients and healthcare workers are educated about the risks and strategies to decrease microbes in the hospital that can cause infection.

If surfaces look dirty, you might think to clean them. But in reality, even surfaces that look clean might harbor microbes. A microbe is a microorganism, especially a bacterium causing disease or fermentation. We sometimes call them germs, bugs or virus. If you have a fear of germs (like me), reading this chapter might make you feel anxious and I have to confess I was anxious talking to Linda. Good news: there are steps you can take to lower your chance of infection. Please read on!

While the likelihood of getting a hospital-acquired infection from a previous patient in the room might be high, with your awareness and some cleaning, you can interrupt the transmission of microbes. Here are some things you need to know:

- There are many surfaces in the hospital room. Look around you. What do you see? Plastic guardrails, bedsheets, pillows, rolling tables made of wood, plastic, or steel. It is important for you to know that not all surface materials can be effectively cleaned or disinfected. This is one reason hand washing is critically important. Watch the behavior of healthcare workers, visitors, and staff, and make note of the surfaces people frequently touch. These are some key areas that must be cleaned.

- Environmental services staff often have just 10 – 15 minutes daily to clean a room, which is not enough time to effectively clean surfaces. As a result, critical areas close to the patient are missed. The cleaning is typically timed, and hospitals have limited environmental services staff. Linda suggests that when you visit your loved one in the hospital, focus on cleaning within three feet of the patient. This typically would include: handrails, nurse call button, rolling bed table, and phone. Make sure staff have provided and keep clean linen. If the patient is able to walk and get out of bed, make sure the sink, faucet and any countertop surfaces in the bathroom are also cleaned regularly.

- Don't assume you know what cleaning products to use on which surfaces – ask. Wipes and cleaners have different chemistry and different uses. Linda shared a story about a woman whose family member had grabbed a washcloth that was on the hospital room counter. She put a little water on the cloth and wiped things down. What she didn't know was that a nursing assistant previously used the washcloth to clean up after a catheter bag filled with urine had spilled. The nursing assistant had used the dry washcloth to wipe the urine off the wall and didn't dispose of it properly in the dirty linen bin. The family member who was trying to be helpful instead contaminated the surfaces she thought she was cleaning.

- Hand washing is key. This actually could be a chapter on its own, as there is a lot to know about hand washing. Linda said that she has done a lot of observational work related to hand washing, and the bottom line is that healthcare workers are good about washing their hands when they enter the patient's room. However, it is what happens next that we should pay attention to. After a healthcare worker uses antibacterial gel or the hand washing station, he or she might then touch the door when closing it, touch their stethoscope (Have they washed it since being used on the last patient?), touch the computer or the IV monitoring system, move the over-bed table, and put down the bedrail. Then, the worker examines or touches the patient. Pay attention to these risks. Hand washing should happen every time before touching the patient.

- Hand washing a patient's hands is also overlooked. Linda shared another story about a patient who was confined to bed for three days. She had an open wound that was draining, and she was attached to many different monitors. The only time staff gave her the opportunity to wash her hands was in the morning during a sponge bath. Not once was she given an opportunity or a way to wash her hands again during the day.

We know that hand washing will interrupt the transmission of microbes. To wash hands properly, use friction for a minimum of 20 seconds, and scrub all surfaces of your hands. This includes in between your fingers, the palms, the back, and around your wrists. It is important to wash hands, encourage others to do it, and make sure the patient is washing hands, especially before eating a meal. Microbes enter the body through the eyes, nose, and mouth. Hand hygiene is critical!

Encouragingly, hospitals are committed to decreasing infection. Let's make it everyone's job to work together towards this goal!

WHY IT MATTERS:

It is important to know that the large majority of healthcare-acquired infections (HAI) are preventable. One in 25 patients has an HAI, meaning that approximately 650,000 people will contract one of these infections annually.[42]

- Healthcare-acquired infections cost the healthcare system and patients billions of dollars annually.

- In American hospitals alone, the Centers for Disease Control and Prevention (CDC) estimates that HAIs account for about 1.7 million infections and 99,000 associated deaths each year. Of these infections, 32 percent of all HAIs are urinary tract infections.

- Those who become infected with HAIs and their families may live completely altered lives due the ongoing care required.

USING THIS INFORMATION:

1. Linda suggests that you ask hospital staff about which cleaning supplies could and should be used on specific surfaces. Some hospitals have video training for family members that discusses the importance of hand hygiene and cleaning surfaces. If this is not available, ask the nursing staff. If the nursing staff cannot tell you how to clean the surfaces, ask to speak with the infection preventionist; every hospital is required to have a director of infection

---

[42] https://psnet.ahrq.gov/primers/primer/7/health-care-associated-infections

prevention on staff. If you still cannot get guidance, go to the administrative office, and ask for someone in patient safety.

2. Know how to properly wash hands: soap and water are best, but even alcohol-based gel is good. You need to wash for a minimum of 20 seconds with friction. Friction is important to remove contamination. Clean between your fingers and all over your hands, including the palms and back of your hands. Wondering how to make sure you do it for a full 20 seconds? Some people sing the birthday song in their head (Happy Birthday to You. Happy Birthday to You. Happy Birthday dear loved one. Happy Birthday to You.).

3. You may feel intimidated to ask healthcare workers and visitors to wash their hands before giving something to the patient or touching the patient. Often the healthcare worker is so focused on patient care they forget to wash their hands again after touching many different surfaces. Linda says that to overcome your fear, remember that if your loved one has an infection, this nurse or doctor will not be living with the health and financial consequences of acquiring an infection – you and your loved one will.

4. If a healthcare worker refuses to wash hands, voice your concern to the head nurse, the hospital patient safety officer, or administration. Linda had an experience with a nurse who refused to wash hands when changing the bandages on a serious wound that was bleeding heavily and many staff were touching. The doctor came in after Linda objected and instructed the nurse to change the wound dressing more frequently. Linda went to administration with her concerns and asked the hospital to not allow this particular nurse to take care of this patient any further. They honored this request. You can ask for that!

SPECIFIC LANGUAGE YOU CAN USE:

- I have been doing a lot of reading and am concerned about risk of infection. Please wash your hands before touching me (or my loved one).

- I am concerned about my wellbeing and know that hospital infection happens. I want to be part of the safety culture here. What products can I use to keep surfaces clean and be helpful in this process?

- Before you touch the patient, please just wash your hands.

- I appreciate that your hospital focuses on safety, and infection is a risk. I would like to help. Which cleaning supplies can I use, and which things should I not touch? (Often sensitive equipment may be part of patient care. This equipment should be cleaned by nursing staff or environmental services. You may ask them to clean those items if they have not been cleaned).

- I would like to help keep the room clean. Where are the supplies for cleaning and which ones should I use on which surfaces?

ADDITIONAL READING AND RESOURCES:

- Kaiser Health News link is a tool which lists hospitals that have been penalized by Medicare for hospital-acquired infection or readmission: https://khn.org/news/hospital-penalties/?penalty=hac

- Review your hospital's safety grade for infection rate and other considerations, assigned by LeapFrog: https://www.hospitalsafetygrade.org/

- CampaignZero's checklist on preventing infections: https://www.campaignzero.org/your-campaignzero-hospital-checklists/help-prevent-c-diff-infections/
- National targets, metrics and progress toward decreasing infections: https://health.gov/hcq/prevent-hai-measures.asp
- Statistics of interest: https://blog.definitivehc.com/statistics-hospital-acquired-conditions
- Hand hygiene fact sheet from the Centers for Disease Control and Prevention: https://www.cdc.gov/features/handhygiene/index.html

ABOUT THE CONTRIBUTOR:

Linda Lybert is CEO of Health Surfaces Consulting and can be reached at linda@healthcaresurfaces.com.

CHAPTER 11

SEPSIS:
1 IN 3 HOSPITAL DEATHS
IS DUE TO SEPSIS

If someone dies in the hospital, the chances are one out of three that it will be because of sepsis, according to the Centers for Disease Control and Prevention (CDC). This chapter is about understanding what sepsis is, how you can identify potential signs of sepsis, and how to stop it from killing you or a loved one.

Mary Millard was a very healthy 55-year-old, retired Licensed Practical Nurse, living out in the country in North Carolina with her husband Mike, before she had an unexpected series of health challenges. Although she and Mike were active, enjoying gardening and walking their dogs, she was experiencing symptoms of A Fib (including irregular, rapid heart rate, fatigue, and shortness of breath). A local health professional prescribed some medicines, which did not help.

When her symptoms became worse, a trip to the emergency room and CT scan (X-ray) revealed that Mary had a 6.5 cm aneurism (which is a ballooning of the heart artery caused by the artery wall weakening) and a partially collapsed aortic valve.

Even though this was a large hospital, Mary was not scheduled for surgery until the following week because the surgeon was out of town. They sent her home to wait.

After four days of feeling worse, she called heart surgeons, in hopes of finding one who could operate right away. She found one after dozens of calls and they admitted her immediately to the hospital where that doctor had hospital privileges and prepped her for surgery. Mary had chosen to get a tissue valve versus a mechanical one, based on her memories of drug side effects she had seen people experience who had chosen mechanical valves. She was clear she didn't want that, and was feeling good about her decision.

She would be ready for surgery in two days. But on the way back from using the bathroom, she said she felt like a dagger was being put through her chest. The hospital staff thought the aneurysm had burst because she was screaming in pain. She remembers seeing her husband Mike holding a folder with their pet pictures he intended to hang in her room. It was the last memory she had of her 65-day ordeal that lay ahead. Another CT scan showed that she had been living with a collapsed heart valve for several days and the pain was likely coming from a clot due to a faulty valve.

In notes put into her medical record that Mary reviewed after her recovery, she read that she coded, meaning she went into cardiac arrest for which the doctors used resuscitative efforts. Nothing worked, and they put her on a machine, called an ECMO, that is life support. It took several days for her to recover to where she could breathe and function enough to be taken off ECMO. The next step according to the notes was getting her ready for open heart surgery. It was urgent because they were afraid the aneurism would burst.

Five days after surgery to fix the aneurism, they moved Mary from intensive care to a step-down unit, which means they were preparing her to go home. However, Mary was not progressing well. She could not get out of bed or squeeze a ball with her hands. She recalls her nurses being frustrated that she wasn't making better, faster progress. One day, Mike noticed that Mary's breathing was strange, and she was talking but making no sense. The nurse believed Mary was having a stroke, which is a common side effect experienced by heart surgery patients.

The nurse called a stroke code, and an eight-hour work up from neurology ensued. In the notes, Mary saw that the neurologist had written, "could this be sepsis?" Unfortunately, it had taken more than a day to determine this – precious time to reverse the sepsis infection before it did further damage.

The hospital called Mike at midnight to come back to the hospital because Mary's organs were shutting down as a response to the sepsis. She was back in ICU and was dying. Mike watched helplessly for days wondering if each one would be Mary's last.

But Mary's immune system was strong, and she was recovering from sepsis. However, two weeks later she needed another surgery to clean out the infection and puss that was filling her chest cavity at the point of surgery. The doctor said this was likely caused by infrequent changing of bandages in her chest sutures. It wouldn't be the last time the hospital failed to detect an infection for various reasons.

In investigating the source of the infection that wracked Mary's body, the hospital believes that the thin tube inserted into Mary's body for the ECMO was likely poised on the edge of the sink in the Cath Lab. As someone washed their hands, it would have been easy for water splashed off the sink drain trap to be the source of contamination. Luckily, Mary ultimately survived with IV antibiotics, although she left the hospital with pseudomonas bacteria. This bug would create its own problems.

Mary spent 20 more days in the step-down unit. She had to learn how to use her hands and walk again. In the course of her surgeries, the hospital staff had ripped her vocal cords, creating hoarseness that caused Mary to speak in whispers.

At home for recovery, Mary received one month of antibiotics by home pump. Mike had to learn how to run a home IV and do physical therapy. Mary went septic again, and her doctor put her on Cipro, a strong antibiotic. During that time, she had some fevers, which her doctors said should be fine because she was taking Cipro. However, at a cardiology appointment, the nurse noticed some sutures which had not been removed, and thought those were probably the cause of Mary's fevers. There was still infection in her body.

Back to the operating room Mary went to have the scarred area cleaned and take the sutures out. While at the ICU, where she was expected to recover for just one night, her heart rate dropped, and she started to get confused. After another culture, it was discovered that the pseudomonas bacteria was back. Mary would be on Cipro tablets for nearly three years.

While Mary's symptoms are now being managed differently, she is committed to helping health professionals and patients understand the risks of hospital infections. She said Mike was scared of hospitals and was not an effective advocate early in her experience. "He went along with the doctor and didn't know the questions to ask … he was shy because of his inexperience with medical issues."

I asked Mary what she wishes she had known or done differently.

Mary believes that nurses and doctors need to be more aware of the symptoms of sepsis and suspect it earlier, because the time to catch sepsis and successfully treat it is short. She regularly speaks with doctors, nurses, and residents to share her story. The symptoms of fever, rapid breathing, and speaking incoherently are not consistent with heart attack and should have been investigated sooner.

Mary said that if Mike could have asked more questions to understand what was happening to her and why, the medical staff may have suspected sepsis sooner. Since Mary has been in and out of the hospital a lot, Mike is now much more comfortable asking questions and is also paying closer attention to Mary's behavior and symptoms.

Mary's top tips, especially for avoiding infection:

- Don't have people bring flowers because there are bacteria in plants and flowers.

- Don't put your silverware on your bed cloth because you can get Clostridium difficile (C. Diff), a bacterium that can cause symptoms ranging from diarrhea to life-threatening inflammation of the colon.

- Ask to have your TV remote, tray table, and surfaces in your hospital room disinfected, or better yet, have a family member take on this task.

ABOUT SEPSIS

When unwanted germs get into a person's body, they can cause an infection. If that infection isn't stopped, it can cause sepsis. According to the CDC, sepsis is the body's extreme response to an infection. It is a life-threatening medical emergency. Sepsis happens when an infection a person already has in the skin, lungs, urinary tract, or somewhere else, triggers a chain reaction throughout the body. Without timely treatment, sepsis can rapidly lead to tissue damage, organ failure, or death.

There are three stages to sepsis. Sepsis can be hard to identify, but typically includes very high or low body temperature, high heart rate, high respiratory rate, high or low white blood cell count, and a known or suspected infection.

EARLY WARNING SIGNS

- fever and chills
- very low body temperature
- urinating less than normal
- rapid pulse
- rapid breathing
- nausea and vomiting
- diarrhea

WHY IT MATTERS:

- According to the Centers for Disease Control and Prevention, it is estimated that sepsis affects around 1.5 million individuals in the United States annually, causing the death of 250,000 individuals and is responsible for one out of every three hospital deaths.[43]
- Time is of the essence! If you suspect sepsis or your loved one has an infection that is not getting better, receiving treatment early can be the difference between surviving or not.

USING THIS INFORMATION:

1. No one test can diagnose sepsis, but when the test results are combined with information about the illness and a physical examination, they can help the doctor decide if

---

[43] https://www.cdc.gov/sepsis/datareports/

the patient has sepsis. Complete blood count (CBC) is a common blood test. There are new blood tests coming out soon that should be able to test proteins in the blood to more rapidly diagnose sepsis.

2. Be aware of the symptoms of sepsis and alert the nurse right away. Make sure to make a note of any unusual behavior in a notebook you keep at the hospital to record information throughout the hospital stay.

3. You can also write the question on the hospital room white board: "Could this be sepsis?" if you can't find someone right away.

SPECIFIC LANGUAGE YOU CAN USE:

- If you suspect sepsis, time is of the essence. Make sure to ask, "Could this possibly be sepsis?"

- Ask for blood tests that can help show blood counts. New tests are coming out to detect specific proteins more rapidly.

- "If this could be sepsis, what action will be taken?" "Which antibiotic will be used, and how will it be delivered?"

- "If we won't know for hours whether or not this is sepsis, what is the risk of getting that antibiotic started sooner? What are the choices?"

- If the patient is not progressing as expected, ask the nurse or doctor, "What do you think is preventing (me/my loved one) from being able to do what is being asked? Could there be something else going on?"

ADDITIONAL READING AND RESOURCES:

- The Sepsis Alliance: https://www.sepsis.org/life-after-sepsis/post-sepsis-syndrome/
- The National Institute of General Medical Sciences sepsis definition: https://www.nigms.nih.gov/education/pages/factsheet_sepsis.aspx
- What is healthcare-acquired infection? https://patientcarelink.org/improving-patient-care/healthcare-acquired-infections-hais/
- How patients can help prevent infections: https://www.cdc.gov/hai/patientsafety/patient-safety.html
- Fact sheets and conversation starters from the CDC: https://www.cdc.gov/sepsis/what-is-sepsis.html

ABOUT THE CONTRIBUTOR:

Mary Millard is currently speaking out nationally about her sepsis experience. To contact Mary, visit: https://marymillard.org.

CHAPTER 12

CARE CONFERENCE: GETTING EVERYONE ON THE SAME PAGE

In thinking about some of the most valuable insider tips I have learned over the years working with advocates, the care conference tops the list. A care conference is a meeting that includes the patient, family, and all professionals who are assisting the patient, with the purpose of getting everyone on the same page in terms of care and decision-making. I didn't know until working in this field that patients and family members can request to be included in a care conference. Care conferences can be critically important, especially in complex cases where doctors from different specialties have differing opinions about how care should proceed. A care conference can take place in the hospital, or in a skilled nursing, or other resident care facility. To help explain how this works, I spoke with Mary Pope, RN, BCPA, who has worked as a health advocate for many years in the Seattle area. Mary shared the story of her client Elliott R.

Elliott was a 74-year old man with type II diabetes and a history of falling. He lived alone with his dog in his Seattle-area home. He occasionally had difficulty walking because of lifelong back problems and previous spinal fusion surgery. A dog walker visited daily to walk his dog, and a neighbor regularly saw Elliott as he walked down his driveway to get the mail. The neighbor noticed over several days that Elliott seemed to have progressively more trouble getting down his driveway. On the fourth day, the dog walker visited Elliott who, by then, could not get up from a seated position. The dog walker and neighbor called a friend, who was a local home health aide to conduct an in-home assessment. Her opinion was that Elliott needed to go to the hospital right away.

At the hospital, his ability to move his arms and legs further declined. Elliott had a lot of tests, including an MRI that showed he had a small stroke, and blood work that revealed a high white blood cell count. However, the medical team believed that the stroke was unrelated to the progressive paralysis he was experiencing. It was unclear what was causing these symptoms.

After two weeks in the hospital Elliot's paralysis seemed to slowly be reversing, and his blood work returned to normal. It was time to begin physical rehabilitation. Elliot was discharged to a skilled nursing facility, which would be a temporary place for him to receive physical therapy and continue to recover and regain mobility.

It was at this point, as Elliott slowly began to regain the use of his arms and legs, that his neighbor contacted health advocate Mary Pope to see if she could help him navigate a new primary care doctor and a series of medical appointments. Mary attended Elliott's first primary care visit and noted that the doctor listened deeply and conducted a very thorough assessment. She also accompanied Elliott to four neurology appointments, where the neurologist was trying to determine the root cause of his paralysis. It was determined, based on his symptoms and tests conducted when Elliot originally went to the hospital, including his increased white blood cell count, that the likely culprit had been a virus.

At skilled nursing facilities, insurance requires regular care conferences, where the whole team meets to discuss the patient's medical and personal needs. Patients and families can attend, but you have to know to ask for it. Although Elliott was generally satisfied with his care in the skilled nursing facility, he had some complaints, and Mary suggested that they participate in a care conference to address his concerns. Because Mary had been working with the social worker on Elliott's behalf, she identified the social worker as the best coordinator for the care conference. The social worker did the scheduling and the facility was very amenable to this meeting. At the care conference, Elliott sat at the head of the table, and team members, including the physical therapist, social worker, and nursing staff participated. Elliot communicated the following issues, with Mary's help:

- He did not feel like the facility staff were treating his pain in a timely or adequate manner.
- He was having trouble sleeping. In the middle of the night he would wake up, and his arm and leg would be numb because he was probably accidentally rolling over and sleeping on his limbs.
- Neuropathic pain (sometimes described as shooting or burning pain) in his legs was not being treated adequately.
- He didn't like the food.
- The person testing his blood sugar was too rough with the finger poker.
- He felt that the safety doors and alarms weren't working.

Mary said that the staff were very professional and used the meeting to brainstorm ideas for improved pain management, food, and other areas of care. They were polite and compassionate despite Elliott's occasional (and understandable) abrasiveness. They acknowledged Elliott's complaints and suggested solutions. Mary noted that while some of these criticisms can seem like minor issues, if unaddressed, especially inadequate pain management, they can become barriers to healing. Elliott wanted to have more control and agency over his recovery, and the facility staff supported this desire.

Elliott and Mary participated in care conferences as his recovery was speeding up and for certain situations where timeliness was important. For instance, Elliott wanted to add an additional physical therapy session to the once-daily session he was receiving. This required coordination with the physical therapist and the facility to determine the out-of-pocket cost to Elliott and whether Medicare covered it. Mary also contacted the doctor (and didn't wait for the care conference to do this) to help understand what Elliott's pain prescription was for and how often he was receiving the pain medicine. She learned that the doctor wrote the prescription so Elliot could only have the pain medicine once a day, in the morning. If he needed it at night, there was no prescription to address that.

Pain medication management is tightly regulated, especially in the face of opioid addiction in our country.[44] In order to receive more pain medicine, Mary scheduled an appointment with Elliott and his new primary care doctor to have a conversation about this. The doctor said that their goal is always to wean people off of pain medication, not to increase it. However, in this situation where Elliott's pain was not being adequately controlled, a temporary increase in medication was reasonable and ordered. In the end, the needed prescription helped his sleep, which was a big part of

---

[44] https://www.drugabuse.gov/drugs-abuse/opioids/opioid-overdose-crisis

Elliott's healing and recovery. He was then able to taper down and eventually eliminate the medicine as his pain subsided. The facility addressed the rest of Elliott's concerns, and he was able to return to his home.

Mary also reflected that for some people care conferences need to happen frequently if communication and care are different than stated expectations.

For instance, another of Mary's clients, a woman named Betty was in a skilled nursing facility and was falling a lot. Surgery had impacted her ability to speak. Betty's family felt like they were not informed enough about her falls. It also concerned them that the facility was not giving her enough attention, especially making sure she ate regularly. Because Betty had difficulty remembering things and could not clearly verbalize her needs, it was challenging for Betty and her family to identify the origin of gaps in her care. It was difficult for Betty to communicate what she was thinking and what she wanted. In this case, a care conference focused on how the team could communicate with the family better and served as a tool to remind the facility that the family was paying attention to her care.

Although Mary's clients were both in skilled nursing, I have seen care conferences used well with patients who are in the hospital or if there is a complicated medical situation where many specialists are involved and have differing opinions about what a patient should do (for instance a choice between surgery, another treatment, or no treatment). It might feel a little daunting for a patient or family member to ask to attend a care conference with multiple doctors, especially if the stakes are high in making a treatment decision that can have life or death consequences. I have seen that hiring and utilizing an advocate to help participate in the care conference and manage the conversation has been very effective.

WHY IT MATTERS:

Doctors may not focus on what matters to patients.[45] In a 2018 survey of more than 2,000 people, patients said that in addition to medical issues, patients wanted to discuss other factors (like sleep, mental health, etc.) that are important to their health.

- In fast-changing or complicated medical situations, it is easy for communication to be imperfect for lots of reasons. Sometimes patients need to make medical decisions quickly. A care conference can get everyone in a room to help make sure all sides of the situation are addressed, and that all parties hear the same information simultaneously.

- It is easy to become emotional or angry if you don't feel like your care, or the care of your loved one is being handled well. Care conferences can also serve to diffuse anger or other emotions, to help understand what is happening, and to mutually and respectfully understand expectations of care.

USING THIS INFORMATION:

1. Family or care team members who can't attend a care conference can send their questions to another participant in advance and can often be included on speaker phone or video conferencing.

2. Be polite even when you're frustrated. The people on the team will inevitably be caring for your loved one when you are not present. Building and maintaining good will

---

[45] https://www.aafp.org/news/practice-professional-issues/20181107doc-patientcomms.html

between the family and caregivers can have a positive impact on the patient's care.

3. When a care conference is requested for a patient who cannot communicate for themselves, it is a good time for the healthcare decision-maker to practice advocating for and communicating decisions on behalf of the patient.

SPECIFIC LANGUAGE YOU CAN USE:

- "What is the Plan of Care?" A Care Plan or Plan of Care is essentially a roadmap to follow, and it is important that you understand what your loved one's Care Plan conveys.

- "We would like to call a care conference to discuss ..." Have your top three issues clearly identified.

- "Help me understand...." Fill in the issue where there may have been a communication disconnect.

- "If (this issue) were to happen again, please walk me through how your facility addresses it, so I understand how you typically manage these situations."

- "Is it possible to ....?" Fill in the blank with communication or procedures you or your loved one would like to happen. By approaching it as a question, you can learn if what you are seeking is even possible.

- If you are screening skilled nursing, assisted living, or hospital facilities for your loved one, you can ask how they handle care conferences. Are they routine? Does the patient or family need to make a request? It is one of many important factors to consider when choosing the right facility for your loved one.

ADDITIONAL READING AND RESOURCES:

- Washington Health Care Association has excellent articles about this topic: https://www.whca.org/directory/all-about-care-conferences/
- Angie's List: How to Prepare for a Home Care Plan: https://www.angieslist.com/articles/how-prepare-nursing-home-care-plan-meeting.htm
- Seattle Children's Hospital description of how care conferences work at their hospital: https://www.seattlechildrens.org/pdf/PE1279.pdf
- Autonomous Care Management has a list of good questions to ask: https://acmcare.org/resident-care-conference/
- Must-Ask Questions for a Nursing Home, from US News and World Report: https://health.usnews.com/health-news/best-nursing-homes/articles/must-ask-questions-when-youre-choosing-a-nursing-home

ABOUT THE CONTRIBUTOR:

Mary Pope, RN, BCPA is an independent health advocate: marytpope@hotmail.com, 425-765-2757. Client information is used with permission.

CHAPTER 13

UNEXPECTED DISCHARGE: THANKS FOR DUMPING MOM

Judy Bloom is a good friend who has spent years working in the field of geriatrics and gerontology services (This focuses on the care of aging people and the study of aging.) Judy's husband is a longtime radiologist in the Seattle area. She is more familiar than most when it comes to understanding the healthcare system. However, Judy was in for an unexpected experience when her mom was hospitalized in 2012 for a fall. Judy learned a lot of lessons about hospital discharge that she wants to share so others will be more prepared and knowledgeable.

In 2012, Judy's mom, Elaine, was 81 years old and living with her husband Abraham, who was wheelchair-bound. They lived in an assisted living apartment, where Abraham had assisted living support and Elaine did not because she was healthy. At the beginning of the week heading into the Thanksgiving holiday, Elaine fell as she attempted to adjust the blinds in their apartment. After the fall she was in a tremendous amount of pain, so the assisted living facility called the emergency medical technicians, and they transported her by ambulance to the hospital. Abraham called Judy, who went immediately to the hospital.

At the hospital, Elaine had many tests to evaluate her pain, including X-rays and a CT scan. She had broken several bones in her spine and was very bruised. Judy was in the hospital with her mom every day and noticed that she couldn't move without significant pain. Elaine was prescribed narcotics and other pain medications to manage her pain, which also made her a risk for falls.

On Thanksgiving Day, with Judy's adult kids and family in town, she called her mom at the hospital to tell her she was on her way to visit, and her mother said that she was being "booted out" immediately, even though she was in terrible pain and couldn't walk on her own.

Without communicating to Judy or giving her any warning, Elaine was put in a cabulance and sent home with a walker. There was no care set up or any evaluation or planning to make sure that someone could care for Elaine on Thanksgiving Day at her apartment. Elaine was met at her apartment by the front desk person who was not a caregiver or someone skilled in transferring people. Judy arrived as soon as possible and began calling caregiving agencies to see if someone could come on Thanksgiving Day and thereafter to provide the care her mom needed.

It was obviously difficult to get services on the holiday for her mom. Judy also had a house full of out-of-town family and guests and was in the midst of cooking. She was pulled in many directions and felt that the hospital just dumped her mom, likely due to having minimal staffing at the hospital on a holiday weekend.

Judy contacted the hospital to express her dissatisfaction with the communications pieces of the discharge for her mom, but that didn't help. Since that time, her parents have had a lot of trips to the hospital for various issues, including more falls and broken bones. One positive improvement that everyone should know about is that there is a new law (Improving Medicare Post-Acute Care Transformation Act of 2014, called the IMPACT Act) that requires hospitals to notify patients covered by Medicare what their rights are regarding discharge from the hospital and how to appeal.

Here is information from the Medicare.gov site:

Within 2 days of your admission and prior to your discharge, you should get a notice called "An *Important Message from Medicare* document about your rights." This notice is sometimes called the Important Message from Medicare or the IM. If you don't get this notice, ask for it. This notice lists the Beneficiary and Family Centered Care Quality Improvement Organization (BFCC-QIO) contact information and explains:

- your right to get all medically necessary hospital services and your right to appeal a decision in the hospital[46]
- your right to be involved in any decisions that the hospital, your doctor, or anyone else makes about your hospital services and to know who will pay for them
- your right to get the services you need after you leave the hospital
- your right to appeal a discharge decision and the steps for appealing the decision
- the circumstances under which you will or won't have to pay for charges for continuing to stay in the hospital
- information on your right to get a detailed notice about why your covered services are ending

---

[46] https://www.medicare.gov/claims-appeals/your-right-to-a-fast-appeal/getting-a-fast-appeal-in-a-hospital#

If the hospital gives you the *Important Message from Medicare* document more than two days before your discharge day, it must do one of these before you're discharged:

- Give you a copy of your original, signed *Important Message from Medicare* document.[47]
- Provide you with a new one that you must sign.

Discharge planning communications often go wrong because there are a lot of coordinating pieces that have to happen from the hospital, including having a doctor ultimately sign paperwork for discharge. I have learned from these experiences:

- Discharge often happens quickly, so you may feel like you are waiting around and then if the orders get signed, there may be a rush to move the patient immediately.
- Hospitals try to discharge patients on Fridays (before a weekend) or before a holiday, because they will have less staff to care for patients.
- Reviewing medicines before you leave and having enough time to purchase medicines before you return home is very important. Often, there are new medicines prescribed or changes to medications. You may have questions about whether certain medicines are needed or not.

---

[47] https://www.medicareadvocacy.org/old-site/InfoByTopic/AcuteHospital/Hospital_07.28.02.IMEnglish.rev.pdf

WHY IT MATTERS:

Being discharged from the hospital can be dangerous. According to the Patient Safety Network:[48]

- 20% of patients discharged from the hospital experience an adverse event within three weeks of discharge that could have been prevented or made better.
- Patients experience drug side effects or complications or hospital-acquired infections.
- 40% of patients are discharged with test results pending, putting patients at risk unless timely and complete follow up is done.
- 20% of Medicare patients are re-hospitalized within 30 days of discharge.

USING THIS INFORMATION:

1. Get a clear plan of the expectations for hospitalization and recovery from the medical team, nursing staff, and social workers.
2. Get a clear and specific idea of what criteria is based upon.
3. Communicate with the place of residence, to get confirmation on what they can and cannot do to support post-hospitalization recovery.
4. If needed, get a backup paid caregiver from a qualified, licensed provider to fill in the gaps of care that will be inevitable.

---

[48] https://psnet.ahrq.gov/primers/primer/11/readmissions-and-adverse-events-after-discharge

5. Be certain that the hospital does not just ship your elderly loved one back home without proper care in place.

6. Make sure that appropriate transport is provided.

7. Insist on the hospital keeping your loved one until all of these specific details are in place.

8. Get help from friends and family.

9. Have an aftercare plan in place to access easily after hospitalization.

10. To figure out how to file a fast appeal to slow down discharge from the hospital go to: https://www.medicare.gov/claims-appeals/your-right-to-a-fast-appeal/getting-a-fast-appeal-in-a-hospital

SPECIFIC LANGUAGE YOU CAN USE:

- I want to appeal this discharge because this will be unsafe for my loved one.

- To help us plan, what will need to happen before discharge?

- My understanding is that the hospital will give us two days' notice before discharge. Can you tell us how this notice will be given to us?

- Who will we be speaking with about discharge to make sure that we have adequate support?

- How do we have a medication review prior to discharge to make sure we know which medicines will be continued, when medicines need to be stopped or tapered, and how the medication list compares to what the patient was taking before hospitalization?

ADDITIONAL READING AND RESOURCES:

- The government's rule on hospital discharge planning: https://www.nhpf.org/library/the-basics/Basics_Hospital-DischargePlanning_02-09-16.pdf
- Research: https://www.elderlawanswers.com/how-medicare-beneficiaries-can-fight-a-hospital-discharge-12218
- Discharge requirements under Medicare: https://www.medicareadvocacy.org/medicare-info/discharge-planning/
- Caregiving: https://www.caring.com/articles/caregiver-organizations
- Medicare Advantage: https://www.medicareinteractive.org/get-answers/medicare-covered-services/hospital-services-inpatient-part-a/your-right-to-hospital-discharge-planning

ABOUT THE CONTRIBUTOR:

Judy Bloom is founder and owner of ThinkWell, LLC, offering executive, leadership development coaching, team engagement facilitation and life cycle coaching. Thinkwellwe.com. She can be reached at Judy@thinkwellwe.com

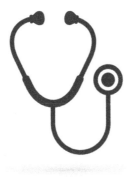

SECTION 4

MONEY MATTERS

SECTION 4

MONEY MATTERS

The business of medicine and healing is expensive. For most of us, costs can be mysterious. Even if we are fortunate enough to have insurance, it is unclear in any given year what we will be paying in total and out of pocket. If we experience an unexpected illness, it can mean a big reduction in our savings.

In thinking about how to approach your healthcare choices, knowing what questions to ask and what health system process is driving tests, procedures and treatment may help inform your decisions. For instance, if you consult a surgeon for surgery, your choices (unless you ask) will focus on surgery and not alternatives.

The healthcare system is set up for efficiency, so if there is a standard of care that is what you will receive, not taking into consideration what you might want or can afford.

ACTION ITEMS:

✓ Use the Drug Prices tool from NeedyMeds to find and compare costs of prescription medicines by zip code: https://www.needymeds.org/drug-pricing

✓ Listen to John Fox's podcast called Medicare Made Simple: https://podcasts.apple.com/us/podcast/medicare-made-simple/id1445616728

✓ Read Consumer Reports article on purchasing medicare supplements: https://www.consumerreports.org/medicare/medicare-advantage-plan/

CHAPTER 14

PRICE TRANSPARENCY AND THE $20 LOTION

I am lucky enough to meet new people regularly who are interested in or curious about health advocacy. Recently, I met with Sarah, a "recovering lawyer" who, over the years, has had a lot of personal experience with health advocacy, for herself, her parents and an older couple whom she helped at the end of their lives because they had no family or friends who could. Her personal story of being charged an extraordinary amount for a small travel-sized lotion while in the hospital and her feelings about it caught my interest, illustrating a larger topic: price transparency.

Sarah and her two sisters are all breast cancer survivors. In 2006 at age 47, she had a mastectomy at a local out-patient hospital in Seattle WA. She had the procedure in a surgical center, limited to performing day surgeries, as it was not a hospital. Fortunately, her insurance, surgical center, hospital and doctors were all part of the same system. She went in for surgery expecting to come home that night (outpatient surgery) or stay just one night for observation.

While the procedure went well, her doctor didn't like the amount of blood that Sarah was losing after surgery, so she was transported by ambulance to the hospital where a second operation took place to try and stop the bleeding. The loss of blood required a blood transfusion, and she stayed in the hospital for several days recovering.

Sarah marveled that there were several things that magically appeared during that short stay, including a toothbrush, toothpaste, and a tiny bottle of hand lotion. No one mentioned them. She didn't ask for them, but she thought it was nice that the nurses were being thoughtful.

After being released from the hospital and recovering nicely at home, Sarah received an itemized bill, which included the price for the tiny lotion (upwards of $20), toothbrush, and toothpaste. Her insurer would not cover these costs, so she called the hospital billing department to say that she didn't ask for these items and that they were outrageously priced. The billing department immediately said those items would be taken off the bill. It left the impression in Sarah's mind that it was unfair to provide items at inflated prices to patients too sick to question the cost. She wondered, "How many people don't question the cost and just pay it?"

Price transparency in healthcare means that the costs are clear to the consumer or patient. The costs of procedures, doctor visits, medicines and medical materials are often difficult to pin down. There are a variety of reasons for this, including that some items are negotiated between the insurer and the provider (the doctor, hospital or organization providing the medical service). Additionally, even if people know the cost of a procedure, for instance, between hospitals, it might not be enough to make a comparative decision on price alone. There are organizations that also evaluate price and value.

As of January 1, 2019, the federal government, through the Department of Health, has issued a policy to help with price transparency. The price transparency rule is overseen by The

Centers for Medicare & Medicaid Services (CMS) which is part of the Department of Health and Human Services (HHS).

Hospitals are required to post their prices in a way that is easy for patients to download. While this will not solve all the challenges patients face in understanding costs related to their care, it is a step forward. As there is more pressure for patients to have more and better understanding of the cost and quality of care, perhaps we will also become more savvy in asking about costs.

WHY IT MATTERS:

- By 2027, one of every five dollars spent in the United States will be spent on healthcare, according to CMS. The impact on individuals and our country's economy is enormous!

- Price transparency not only serves an educational purpose, it actually lowers the cost of healthcare. According to an article in *Health Affairs*, both price transparency and reference pricing — the cost consumers can anticipate paying for a given procedure or health service — have helped reduce costs in the long run.[49]

- Requesting items in the hospital can be unnecessarily costly.

USING THIS INFORMATION:

1. Price transparency itself is not a goal. It is a means toward multiple goals including helping patients avoid sticker shock, facilitating shopping, lifting the veil on high prices, and ultimately making care more affordable.[50]

---

[49] https://www.healthaffairs.org/do/10.1377/hblog20150707.049155/full/
[50] https://catalyst.nejm.org/how-to-teach-people-about-health-care-pricing/

2. For planned procedures, call ahead to your medical provider and have a conversation about the procedure, billing codes and what (if anything) people having the same procedure have had questions about.

3. The Centers for Medicare & Medicaid Services (CMS), which is part of the federal government's Department of Health implemented a rule as of January 1, 2019 requiring hospitals to post the costs of services and items that they charge for on their website in a format you can easily access. If you don't find it easily, call the billing department and ask to be directed to the specific URL.

SPECIFIC LANGUAGE YOU CAN USE (WITH THE INSURER):

- What are the billing codes or names of items I need to know to determine the costs I might anticipate? What is the formulary used to determine the cost? (A formulary is a list of prescription drugs that are covered by a specific health care plan. A formulary can contain both name-brand and generic drugs. Patients pay co-pays on formulary drugs. If a drug is not on the list, the patient will pay much more, up to the full cost of the drug.)

- Will my insurance cover specific costs? What will I likely pay out of pocket?

ADDITIONAL READING AND RESOURCES:

- "How Price Transparency Can Control the Cost of Health Care" https://www.rwjf.org/en/library/research/2016/03/how-price-transparency-controls-health-care-cost.html

- In Washington state, use the WAhealthcomare.com website, a tool to compare the costs of procedures: https://www.wahealthcarecompare.com/

- Going above the price transparency rule: https://revcycleintelligence.com/features/going-above-and-beyond-the-cms-hospital-price-transparency-rule

- Goals for price transparency and how to measure its success: https://catalyst.nejm.org/health-care-price-transparency-goals/

ABOUT THE CONTRIBUTOR:

Sarah Hopkins is the Regional Health Administrator for Public Health in Seattle.

CHAPTER 15

COMPARISON SHOPPING CAN PAY OFF

I met Judy Cushman in the early 1990s when I was working at the biotechnology company, Immunex. She worked in executive search for biotechnology and other corporate clients in the Seattle area and nationally. We recently reconnected after her sister's death when Judy developed an interest in the field of health advocacy. She shared a recent personal story about an eye procedure that she had, pointing out that even a savvy, intelligent, engaged patient like she is, can learn additional questions to ask before a potentially costly surgery. What she didn't know beforehand was that when you pick certain doctors or locations for surgery, the cost can vary extraordinarily.

Judy was seen by her regular eye doctor for a scheduled routine exam. Her doctor mentioned that Judy had spots or floaters in her eyes. It was not a dangerous condition, but it impaired her vision. Her doctor recommended a retinal specialist group and gave her their card. Having always been proactive about her health, Judy said she had absolutely no fear about asking questions. She considered herself far more informed than most people about health matters. She followed up and made an appointment, initially knowing very little about this specialized practice area. So, in advance of her first retinal eye appointment, she asked:

- "Do I need a driver?" (yes)
- "Will the doctor be dilating my eyes?" (yes)
- "How long will the appointment be?" (half day)
- "Will my insurance cover the appointment charge?" (yes)

In addition to the extensive tests, the eye specialist asked her a number of questions about how impactful the floaters in her eye were, and Judy answered the questions honestly. The specialist told her the good news that she qualified for vitrectomy surgery. The surgery would replace the fluid in the eye, remove the floaters, and "clean up" the lens in her eye.

The next step was to line Judy up for the hospital where the specialist operated. The specialist said that they chose a specific hospital because they had the best equipment and the most up to date services. Judy assumed that the hospital was in-network and therefore covered by her insurance because both the original doctor and the specialist were covered by her insurer. She agreed to the procedure.

However, two weeks before she was due to be at the hospital, her retinal eye doctor's nurse called Judy and said that the hospital for the surgery was out of the network. In this case, her surgery would not be eligible for a negotiated rate. She would have to pay 50% of the $20,000 surgery. Judy decided to not have the surgery. $10,000 was too expensive!

Judy was determined to find another eye surgeon who could perform the surgery in-network. She called her regular healthcare provider who was in-network and determined they had specialists who could perform the surgery. She went through the entire set of tests again. Her eyes were again dilated. This took a half day as before. She assumed, since she had qualified to have the procedure previously that she would be qualified with a new doctor. Even with the same exam, the second doctor, who was admittedly very conservative, said she would only perform the procedure if Judy were virtually blind. The doctor felt she was borderline and therefore would not offer her the procedure. The doctor recommended she seek another opinion.

Frustrated that she had spent so much time without resolution, Judy researched other specialists and found one that did nothing but retinal surgeries. The specialist group happened to be 15 minutes from her home. This time before her exam, the specialist sent a note about what to expect from the exam. The office said that her eyes would be dilated, she would need a driver, etc. Although she was not happy about going through three exams of the same type of tests for the same problem, she was impressed with this specialist's practice.

They told Judy that she did qualify for the procedure and the cost to her was 15% of the negotiated in-network cost, which equaled about $600 out of pocket. However, they also noted that they contract out for anesthesia, which is not unusual. She tracked down the anesthesiologist to ask what the cost would be. Fortunately, the anesthesiologist, although contracted, was in-network and covered by her insurance. At least she wouldn't be surprised by the costs.

If Judy hadn't been told that the original specialist was out of network, she would have had to pay $10,000. Judy summarizes what she learned from this experience in the "Using this information section" below.

WHY IT MATTERS:

- The cost of healthcare is now Americans' top financial concern, according to a Gallup Poll.[51]

- The cost of out of pocket expenses has increased by more than 41 percent between 2010 and 2014,[52] and more costs are being shifted to patients.

- There is wide variability in costs for the same procedure, and patients believe that comparison shopping is important, but few people actually do it. In a study published in *Health Affairs*, only 13% of respondents sought information about expected costs before receiving care, and only 3% compared costs of providers before receiving care.[53] Checking the costs can save you thousands of dollars!

- Sometimes it matters where you have your test, procedure, or surgery.

USING THIS INFORMATION:

1. Don't assume that just because your doctor has the card of a specialist that your doctor actually knows the specialist well. You can ask your doctor if they recommend the doctor; if your doctor knows the specialist; and if there are any cross-referral fees associated.

---

[51] https://news.gallup.com/poll/212780/cost-healthcare-americans-top-financial-concern.aspx

[52] Bloche MG. Consumer-directed healthcare. N Engl J Med. 2006; 355 (17): 1756 – 9. Crossref, Medline, Google Scholar

[53] https://www.healthaffairs.org/doi/full/10.1377/hlthaff.2016.1471

2. Make sure to understand before your appointment, procedure or visit, if your insurance will cover it. Like in Judy's case, sometimes you have to research the provider to check first.

3. Always ask how long the appointment or procedure will be, so you will be prepared. Unlike a normal business appointment where you typically have a scheduled amount of time agreed to in advance, patients don't always ask this important question.

SPECIFIC LANGUAGE YOU CAN USE:

- What are all the costs associated with this test/procedure/visit/hospitalization?
- Are these costs covered by my insurance, and what will I be responsible for?
- Is the referral you are providing someone you know well? Are there any financial incentives in place for this referral?
- I plan to seek a second opinion; please provide my records so I understand the tests and opinion you have provided. I would like to come back to discuss my options.
- Are there options for where to have this procedure? Do they vary in cost?
- Are there any contracted medical personnel (like anesthesiologists) who are not covered in the cost estimate you provided?

ADDITIONAL READING AND RESOURCES:

- Leapfrog is an online resource to help you choose the best hospital and doctor using price transparency and quality tools: https://www.leapfroggroup.org/compare-hospitals

- Medicare.gov has a site called Hospital Compare: https://www.medicare.gov/hospitalcompare/search.html?

- Cost comparison tools: http://www.truthinhealthcare.org/consumer-resources/cost-comparison-tools/

CHAPTER 16

FINANCIAL TOXICITY

Dana Hutson is a health advocate on the east coast who specializes in providing clarity to the confusion of a cancer diagnosis. I met Dana several years ago as she was launching her business and was impressed with her practical, authentic, and credible approach to helping patients. I had never heard of the concept of financial toxicity – meaning the financial side effects of cancer treatment can be as devastating as the physical ones. Dana shared a story of a friend, colleague and eventual client who, despite her financial literacy, suffered the silent side effects of financial toxicity.

At a DC-area Chamber of Commerce meeting in 2014, Dana and her colleague Jemma met while listening to Carly Fiorina, former Hewlett-Packard CEO speak. Jemma would also work with Dana through various business organizations, including the local Women Business Owners organization. Dana knew Jemma as a smart, resilient, caring, and successful wealth manager in her 60s who had built a thriving practice. She was an exceptional planner, not only in finance but in life. In fact, Jemma's life motto was, "Life Happens. Be Ready." Jemma's goal was to sell her very successful business when she retired, leave a financial nest egg for her children, and enjoy traveling with her husband and grandchildren.

As a wealth manager, Jemma was more savvy than most about money, but discussing personal money matters, especially for women, is still the exception rather than the norm. So, it was surprising to Dana when Jemma confided to her in 2016 that she had been diagnosed with advanced breast cancer and she needed help. Dana would work with her as a friend and toward the end of her disease as a client helping her family sort out her medical and end of life decisions.

Dana had heard about the concept of financial toxicity in 2004 from a cancer specialist who was a pioneer in utilizing innovative specialty immunotherapies that were very effective, however at an expense never seen by patients before. This doctor told Dana that he was very satisfied with the therapy, which caused almost no side effects and was extremely effective, however it caused substantial "green-openia" – an unprecedented financial impact on his patients. Today, innovative immunotherapies are commonplace, and the cost of innovation is not cheap.

Although she had good insurance, over the course of her cancer journey, Jemma pursued clinical trials and complementary treatments throughout the country, incurring costly out of pocket expenses. This is a common situation due to the increased cost of healthcare innovation and the insurance companies' practice of cost sharing, where a larger proportion of costs is shifted to the patients. The result is higher out of pocket expenses for patients who are paying higher deductibles, plus increases in co-pays and co-insurance. Even people with good insurance often find themselves underinsured.

Treatments and her disease took their toll on her business. Jemma was unable to keep up with her work schedule which resulted in a loss of income – another aspect of the financial toxicity of treatment. Jemma had planned to sell a healthy business, but instead the fruit of decades of business building was spent on the cost of treatment. Her dream of selling a thriving business was dashed. Eventually Jemma had to shutter the doors and close her business.

Dana said that Jemma also felt a little ashamed because she had built a wealth management business only to have her dreams thwarted by the financial toxicity of her illness. Although she had good insurance and didn't go into bankruptcy, the unforeseen financial effects of managing her cancer caused distress and embarrassment. Could she have had a different financial outcome?

When Dana started to help her, it was too late to apply some of the strategies that would have assisted with many of the previously incurred out of pocket expenses. With research, Dana identified many areas where costs could have been saved if Jemma had only known this was a potential side effect of her treatment and addressed this financial issue with her healthcare team earlier in her disease management journey.

Had Jemma, who was a planner, been aware of the out of pocket expenses she would incur, she would have been prepared.

WHY IT MATTERS:

- According to the National Cancer Institute (NCI), financial toxicity is more likely to happen to cancer patients.[54]
- NCI also makes the following key points after studying this issue:[55]
  - Patients may not take their medicine as directed so that they can save money on copayments.
  - Patients experiencing financial toxicity may have a lower quality of life.

---

[54] https://www.cancer.gov/publications/dictionaries/cancer-terms/def/financial-toxicity
[55] https://www.cancer.gov/about-cancer/managing-care/track-care-costs/financial-toxicity-pdq

○ Financial toxicity at its worst can lead to debt and bankruptcy.

- Other studies have shown that financial toxicity is associated with depression and anxiety.[56]

- The financial pressure of healthcare is real. In a 2018 survey for the Commonwealth Fund, respondents reported:[57]

    ○ More than a third of seriously ill patients are not confident they can afford their healthcare costs if faced with a dire financial situation.

    ○ More than half have experienced severe financial hardships related to their care.

    ○ Almost a quarter were unable to pay for things like food, heat, and housing.

USING THIS INFORMATION:

1. The National Cancer Institute provides synonyms to financial toxicity such as economic burden, economic hardship, financial distress, financial hardship, and financial stress.

2. The best time to think about potential financial distress is before you face a medical experience. Some things to consider are your overall debt and savings. If you have access to a financial planner, wealth manager, or financial counselor, it is a good idea to speak with them about strategies to help you understand what the financial implications for your situation might be.

3. The cost of innovative medicine or treatment can be expensive and even good insurance may require you to pay more

---

[56] https://ascopubs.org/doi/abs/10.1200/JCO.2018.36.15_suppl.e22037
[57] http://features.commonwealthfund.org/health-care-in-america

than you can afford. Pharmaceutical companies often have financial assistance programs to help you afford your treatment. You can typically apply for these programs by contacting the company and filling out an application. Your doctor will likely also need to provide information and paperwork. If you qualify, you may be able to obtain your medicine for free.

4. If your child is sick with a qualifying disease, including cancer, he or she may be eligible to be treated at St. Jude Children's Research Hospital. St. Jude's provides treatment without charging patients who fall within the treatment categories they have identified. www.stjude.org

5. The best thing you can do is be proactive and start the conversation.

SPECIFIC LANGUAGE YOU CAN USE:

The Hospital or Doctor

- Whom can I speak with regarding the financing of my treatment? (at the hospital/doctor/institution) I need to understand all the aspects of this treatment. Can you identify what is being suggested, what all the costs will be, and who I can speak with about the priorities for treatment?

The Pharmaceutical Company or Manufacturer

- Do you have a patient assistance program that may help me pay for my medicines or treatment, or help me get the medicines or treatment at a reduced cost?

- What are the qualification criteria to be covered by the patient assistance or other program you may have to help me afford my medicine or treatment?

ADDITIONAL READING AND RESOURCES:

- RIP Medical Debt is a 501(c)(3) charity that has abolished $635 million in medical debt for more than 200,000 Americans. To donate ($100 donation forgives $10,000 in debt), or to access this information, go to their website: https://www.ripmedicaldebt.org/about/

- There are many organizations that may offer grants to cover the cost of medical travel. Organizations include: Air Charity Network, Miracle Flights, National Patient Travel Center, Patient AirLift Services, and the American Cancer Society.

Help Paying for Medicines:

- NeedyMeds is a national nonprofit organization that maintains a website of free information on programs that help people who can't afford medications and healthcare costs. www.needymeds.org, or call their helpline at 800.503.6897.

- Partnership for Prescription Assistance: A program sponsored by drug companies, doctors, patient advocacy organizations, and civic groups, helps low-income, uninsured patients get free or low-cost, brand-name medications.

- RxAssist: An online database of drug company programs that provide free or affordable drugs and co-pay assistance.

- Center for Benefits: Provided by the National Council on Aging, this shares information about assistance programs for low-income seniors and young people with disabilities. https://www.ncoa.org/centerforbenefits/

- RxHope: A web-based resource where you can search by medication to locate assistance programs. They also offer help with the application process https://www.rxhope.com/.

- RxOutreach: A mail-order pharmacy for people with little to no health insurance coverage https://rxoutreach.org/ and what you might want to know from WebMD: https://www.webmd.com/health-insurance/mandated-to-buy-insurance

- Patient Assistance Foundation: https://www.copays.org/

- The Cancer Financial Assistance Coalition (CFAC) is a group of national organizations that provide financial help to patients. CFAC provides a searchable database of financial resources: https://www.cancerfac.org

- "The Financial Toxicity of Illness" https://www.nytimes.com/2019/02/21/well/live/the-financial-toxicity-of-illness.html

ABOUT THE CONTRIBUTOR:

Dana Hutson is founder and president of Cancer Champions and can be reached at https://cancer-champions.com/. Her friend's story is used with her permission.

CHAPTER 17

UNDERSTANDING MEDICARE: DEMYSTIFYING YOUR CHOICES

John Fox is a family man who moved to Spokane, WA to be closer to his adult daughters and grandkids after a successful business career in financial management and insurance. In addition to his volunteer work and his woodworking, he runs a business called We Speak Medicare, which helps people understand how to select the best options for Medicare Insurance. I have been fortunate to know John through his work on the Washington State Health Advocacy Board (www.washaa.org).

Although I am constantly learning something from John – about work or life – I thought his experience in helping people make their Medicare choices might be helpful in understanding that there are people and organizations that can help ordinary people make better choices. We Speak Medicare helps people find programs that align with a person's circumstances and specific needs. You have to know how to ask and where to look.

Before you turn 65 and are eligible for Medicare, you will receive a booklet called, *Medicare & You*. This booklet has everything you need to know about Medicare and the choices you need to make. John remarked that most people are very confused because there is a lot of information that pertains to just a few people, not everyone.

Medicare is a federal program that provides health insurance to people who are age 65 and older, blind, or disabled. Medicare consists of four parts:

- **Part A** pays for hospital care.
- **Part B** provides medical insurance for doctor's fees and other medical services.
- **Part C** is Medicare Advantage, which allows beneficiaries to enroll in private health plans to receive Part A and Part B Medicare benefits.
- **Part D** covers prescription drugs.

If you are receiving social security benefits, you will automatically be enrolled in Part A at no additional cost once you turn 65. If you do not receive social security benefits, you will need to enroll in Part A as early as three months before your 65th birthday. Parts B, C, and D are voluntary and require people to pay premiums to receive coverage specific to that part.

John said that it is important to know that you will pay the same rate for Medicare whether you purchase Supplemental Plans for Parts B, C or D through an insurance company, an insurance broker, or through your company, as some employers subsidize this cost. Medicare authorizes different plans with various benefits through many insurance companies. Each plan may be different depending on how you pay (Premiums are set monthly payments; deductibles are payments you agree to make for certain services, and out of pocket costs are those that you are responsible for.). It is important to look at your needs to determine the right plan including the total amount you might pay and whether you need coverage for prescription medicines. For instance, if you have a chronic condition like diabetes or rheumatoid arthritis, this may impact your needs for supplemental insurance.

An insurance broker that sells supplemental Medicare through many different insurance companies might have the best knowledge to help a specific individual, because they can compare each plan for you. An agent that just represents one insurance company may not know about what other plans have to offer. It is important to know how many and which insurance plans the agent is licensed to sell. Agents are required by the federal government (through the Department of Health/Centers for Medicare and Medicaid Services, called CMS) to take and pass an annual exam for each plan and insurance company they sell.

In Washington State, there is a program called SHIBA, Statewide Health Insurance Benefits Advisors. SHIBA provides free, unbiased and confidential assistance with Medicare and health choices through trained volunteers.

Nationally, the Patient Advocate Foundation (PAF) is a national 501 (c)(3) non profit organization which provides case management services and financial aid to Americans with chronic, life threatening and debilitating illnesses. Organization materials and case managers can be reached through the website at: https://www.patientadvocate.org/

In order to find a reliable Medicare agent, John suggests you talk to your estate planning attorney, or eldercare attorney whom you trust. Another good source might be a financial planner. Building a relationship with your advocate team for health should include someone who can help you with insurance choices, regardless of wether you are on Medicare or another insurance coverage.

John shared a story with me about a gentleman who contacted him because he received a bill from a local hospital that was almost $200,000. The hospital said that Medicare had declined coverage because he didn't qualify. After John asked him some questions about his situation and knew that Medicare generally covered the reason for his hospital stay, John felt like it didn't sound correct that Medicare would deny coverage. It isn't always clear to someone who doesn't deal with Medicare on a regular basis exactly what is covered in every situation.

John and the gentleman initiated a three-way call with the hospital and then conferenced in the Medicare phone representative directly to ask the reason why the hospital charges were declined. As it turned out, the hospital had not provided enough information for Medicare to determine whether he qualified for the surgery. Medicare needed to understand why he had the surgery.

Once that was settled, John asked if the hospital provided an advance beneficiary notice to let the man know his hospital expenses might not be covered. The advance beneficiary notice is provided by the hospital if they believe for any reason your charges might not be covered by Medicare. As it turned out the hospital had not provided an advance beneficiary notice. If the hospital does not provide this, patients are not responsible for the charges.

WHY IT MATTERS:

- According to AARP, there are 44 million people (15% of the US population) enrolled in Medicare, and that number is expected to rise to 79 million by 2030.[58]

- Medicare represents 14 percent of all federal spending in the United States, pays for one-fifth of all healthcare spending, and is the second largest program in the federal budget.[59]

- If you don't choose your Medicare options or insurance wisely, you could be overpaying.

---

[58] https://assets.aarp.org/rgcenter/health/fs149_medicare.pdf
[59] https://www.pgpf.org/budget-basics/medicare#footnote1

- There is a lot to know about Medicare, so having a trusted agent or advisor can help you make sure you are selecting the right supplements to meet your needs.

USING THIS INFORMATION:

1. When selecting any insurance coverage, you should have a list of your prescription medicines, your general health history, and an understanding of your financial situation so you can weigh the pros and cons of plans that have up front expenses (premiums and high deductibles) vs. high out of pocket or catastrophic costs.

2. Do you go to the hospital frequently? Do you have an ongoing medical condition that requires continual care?

SPECIFIC LANGUAGE YOU CAN USE WITH AN AGENT:

- Which insurance companies and Medicare plans are you licensed to sell?
- If I have high cost prescription medicines, what is my best plan for Medicare Part D? Are there other supplements I should consider?
- What is my portion of costs for services and supplies?
- How will my providers be covered or not by the network designated in the plan? Can I still see my provider if they are not part of the network? Will it cost extra for me?
- Does the plan offer benefits Medicare doesn't cover, like vision, hearing, dental, or prescription drug coverage (different than Part D Plan)?

ADDITIONAL READING AND RESOURCES:

- The Resource Center for Medicare: https://www.cms.gov/About-CMS/Agency-Information/OMH/resource-center/index.html

- United Healthcare overview on Medicare: https://www.medicaremadeclear.com/

- AARP Guide to Medicare: https://www.aarp.org/health/medicare-insurance/info-2018/medicare-made-easy.html

ABOUT THE CONTRIBUTOR:

John Fox is founder of We Speak Medicare. John can be reached at johnfoxtsp@gmail.com or 509-990-1886. https://wespeakmedicarespokane.com/

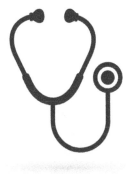

SECTION 5

THE ADVOCATE
BY YOUR SIDE

THE ADVOCATE BY YOUR SIDE

It might seem obvious that a patient can benefit from having an advocate, but what does that mean? Although nurses have traditionally fulfilled the role of advocating on behalf of the patient, as the healthcare system has evolved to greater efficiency, the role of nurses has changed. Nursing staff shortages, increasing electronic charting, and narrowing the role of nurses in hospitals have impacted what patients can expect from nurses.

Patients benefit from having an extra person speak on their behalf. This is often a family member. Patients who happen to have family who are nurses or doctors have an inside track to potentially better care due to that person's understanding of how the system works in addition to understanding medical aspects of care.

An advocate can be defined in many ways but is generally someone who can speak on behalf of the patient to help the patient have more choice and control in medical decision-making. The field of health and patient advocacy is still relatively new. In the past ten years, the number of people practicing as independent health and patient advocates has increased. This role includes aging life care consultants and a wide variety of individuals or companies that work directly for the patient.

There are several courses that advocates can take to help them learn about this role. Aging Life Care practitioners have several certifications, and in 2017, the Patient Advocate Certification Board launched the Certified Patient Advocate credential. However, patients should understand that these certifications are independent and separate from medical organizations such as the American Medical Association.

While family members and friends may be a good choice for many patients, there are advantages to having an independent advocate. This person:

- is a neutral navigator, someone who works for the patient without any other obligation or motivation
- may have a specific expertise (i.e., insurance, specific disease area, hospital expertise, etc.)
- can speak the medical lingo
- may have connections with outside resources, such as personally know the doctors in the area or how specific hospitals or practices handle cases

FOR FURTHER LEARNING:

- ✓ If you want to become a Patient Advocate, you can take the following course and exam: https://pacboard.org/exam/
- ✓ Participate in Family Patient Advocate Training in New York: https://pulsecenterforpatientsafety.org/fcpa-class/
- ✓ Take a Patient Advocacy Class in California: https://empoweredpatientcoalition.org/training/workshops/
- ✓ Attend one of the following: Patient Know More!, The Volunteer Health Advocate Training Program, or the Emerging Field of Health Advocacy Presentations by a

WASHAA representative: http://www.washaa.org/request-a-presentation.html

ACTION ITEMS:

✓ Identify who would make an ideal advocate and consider:
- your trust in them
- his or her personality
- their reliability
- geographic proximity/availability
- interest in helping

✓ Identify and name your Health Care Proxy, and fill out a Durable Power of Attorney for Health Care to make sure you have someone to make decisions for you in case you cannot.

✓ If you are interested in finding an independent advocate in your geographic area or with specific expertise, you can find advocates on the following directories:
- Aging Life Care Association: https://www.aginglifecare.org/
- Alliance of Professional Health Advocates https://aphadvocates.org/
- Greater National Advocates (broken up by geographic area):
  - Greater Chicago Advocates: http://chicagoadvocates.com/
  - Greater Southwest Advocates: http://greatersouthwestadvocates.org/
  - Greater West Advocates: http://greaterwestadvocates.org/

- National Association of Healthcare Advocacy https://www.nahac.com/
- Washington State Health Advocates Association www.washaa.org

CHAPTER 18

HOME CARE HELP:
DIFFERENT FROM HOME HEALTH CARE

Shawn D'Amelio is the Director of Business Development for a home care company called With a Little Help, in the Greater Seattle area. I have known her for about a decade through our work in the health advocacy field. She is the president of the Washington Home Care Association, which helps people find licensed home care agencies.

As we know, language matters and people often confuse home care and home health. Home health is ordered by a physician and paid by Medicare (if approved) or is paid privately. Home health is performed by a nurse, social worker or therapist for a period of up to 60 days for those who cannot leave the home due to their health status. Shawn observes that it is an underutilized benefit and it is your right to request your doctor to order it for you to help you build strength and prevent hospitalization.

Home health is often ordered at the time of discharge from a hospital or skilled nursing community and can include the following:

- visiting nurse

- social worker
- physical therapy
- speech therapy
- ostomy care
- intravenous therapy
- medication
- wound care

Home care, however, is NOT physician-ordered and is not reimbursed by Medicare at this time but will be soon. Some long term care insurance, Veteran's benefits or Medicaid will cover the costs if you need assistance with activities of daily living (eating, bathing, dressing, toileting, transferring). Home caregivers can help with a variety of things, depending on the patient's needs:

- grocery shopping & errands
- meal preparation
- companionship
- transportation
- pet walking and care
- personal care (bathing and dressing)
- toileting and incontinence care
- respite for family
- light housekeeping
- medication reminders
- assistance with exercise
- management of chronic conditions
- nurse delegating care (helping to take medicines)

When I asked Shawn how families know when hiring a home caregiver might be important, she said to look for a decline in appearance, isolation, bruising, weight loss, falls, missed appointments, stacks of bills, overdue payment notices, missed medications, or multiple hospitalizations. Home caregivers serve as advocates because they work alongside the client and family to provide patient centered care, assure medication compliance, good nutrition, engagement and assistance with activities of daily living. Caregivers can be a second set of eyes to observe the needs and behaviors of a loved one for a family member who doesn't live close by, works, or has children to care for as well.

Shawn shared a story about one of her clients, Pearl. Pearl was the eighty-year-old mother of two children who were doctors. The children were concerned about their mom because they were noticing more memory issues, so they thought it might be a good idea to evaluate whether a part-time caregiver was enough help, or if they needed to bring in more care. What they learned when Shawn met their mom in her home was startling to them.

First, Pearl kept her 10 – 15 medication packets in the bathroom all together. Shawn asked if Pearl could show her which medications she had taken that morning. To the children's surprise Pearl was not able to do that.

Shawn set up a medications management system called a Mediset. A Mediset is a special medication container that gives visual and audio cues when it is time to take your medication. It is pre-filled by family members or a pharmacist with all medications required for the week, bi-weekly or month depending on how often you take medication. Pearl couldn't even manage that. It was a clear message, Shawn said, for them to understand their mom needed a different and higher level of care than her sons had originally thought.

Also, on that visit, Shawn asked Pearl to sit on the toilet (with clothing on) to show Shawn how she arose from the toilet. There were no grab bars and Pearl was unsteady, so she used the towel bar to get up. After the evaluation, Shawn recommended adding a toilet seat with handles to make it easier to get up. Pearl's sons had no idea that she was having challenges getting up from a chair and the toilet until the home care visit from Shawn.

Shawn has seen the benefits of caregiving in the lives of her clients. She said that one of the goals of having a caregiver is to allow aging loved ones to stay independent and live in their own home, if that is what they wish. Shawn says that when caregivers assist with nutrition, medication compliance, exercise, engagement, hygiene and transportation for groceries and appointments, something wonderful happens . . . friendships bloom and there are fewer trips to the ER due to illness, falls, and infection.

Shawn said that not all caregivers are the same, and people should be careful of hiring unlicensed caregivers. These types of caregivers are often found on Craigslist or through websites that compile unlicensed and unsupervised caregivers.

Licensed home care agencies perform background checks, fingerprinting, conduct formal training, have back up caregivers, provide supervision, pay payroll taxes and also provide benefits to their caregivers. Shawn warns that when hiring unlicensed caregivers, you are essentially responsible for complying legally as the employer. That means you must know and follow the law with regard to payroll taxes, worker's compensation, reference checks, minimum rest breaks, as well as carefully managing the caregiver's schedule to not exceed the maximum number of hours worked, etc.

The risks, Shawn says, are many. Crimes against seniors are higher than ever and hiring a licensed and bonded home care company is one way to protect them. Shawn shared a story about meeting with lawmakers in Olympia, WA to discuss issues related to home care, hospice and palliative care. One of the home care owners shared that he had received a call from a man who hired a caregiver off of Craigslist who had stolen $5,000 from the client. Although he assisted the man to file a police report, the man was unable to reclaim the money that was taken.

Another sign that caregiving is needed is if a loved one has lost the ability to know what to do in an emergency. Shawn related how one client had fallen in the middle of the night and lay on the floor without calling 911, because she didn't want the siren to disturb the neighbors.

People who want to be proactive can plan to have support in the home before they might need it urgently. Shawn suggests that families should and can start by identifying a licensed home care agency they feel comfortable with and then interview them. Families can initially start by hiring someone for just a couple of hours a week in order to begin building a relationship. Home caregivers can be hired to go anywhere: independent living, assisted living, memory care, or adult family home.

WHY IT MATTERS:

- Of the older adults who were living outside nursing homes or hospitals in 2010, nearly one third (11.3 million) lived alone, according to the Institute on Aging.[60]
- Many older people who live alone say they feel lonely and isolated.

---

[60] https://www.merckmanuals.com/home/older-people%E2%80%99s-health-issues/social-issues-affecting-older-people/older-people-living-alone

- Because eating is a social activity for most people, some older people who live alone do not prepare full, balanced meals. Thus, undernutrition becomes a concern.

- Among people with health problems or difficulty seeing or hearing, it is all too easy for new or worsening symptoms of disease to go unnoticed.

- Many older people who live alone have problems following directions for prescribed treatments, which can lead to up to 75% of older adults making medication errors resulting in severe side effects, hospitalization or worse.

USING THIS INFORMATION:

Shawn says that there are a few signs to look for that may indicate it is time to hire a caregiver:

1. Is your loved one falling?
2. Do you see bruises?
3. Are they spending a lot of time alone?
4. Is their appearance declining?
5. Are they losing weight?
6. Are bills piling up on the counter – or maybe there are late bill notices?
7. Is your loved one missing appointments?
8. If your loved one has a mobile "HELP" button, do they know how to activate it and receive help?
9. Are they having difficulty remembering how they would dial 911 if they fell, and would they be willing to dial it if needed?

SPECIFIC LANGUAGE YOU CAN USE:

What to ask potential caregivers before you hire them:

- Are you licensed? Is the company you work for licensed?
- Are you bonded and insured? If so, may I see your insurance?
- Who pays for your Worker's Compensation and taxes?
- Who will cover your shift if you are sick?
- What kind of training do you have?
- Do you have a background check from your company, or may I run a background check?
- May I talk to a reference – someone you have worked for?

In evaluating if your loved one needs help, you can say:

- Show me what medicines you took this morning/afternoon/evening. (to make sure they can keep medicines straight)
- Can you show me how you would get up from the toilet/fix a meal/follow instructions?
- If you smelled smoke, what would you do?
- What happened to cause that bruise?
- What are your goals?

ADDITIONAL READING AND RESOURCES:

- Tips on Choosing a Caregiver: https://blog.ioaging.org/caregiving/tips-on-choosing-the-right-caregiver-for-an-older-loved-one/

- AARP How to Hire a Caregiver: https://www.aarp.org/caregiving/home-care/info-2018/hiring-caregiver.html
- 50 Mistakes to Avoid When Selecting Home Care Services: https://blog.caregiverhomes.com/50-mistakes-to-avoid
- Washington Home Care Association: https://wahca.org/
- National Association of Home Care & Hospice: https://www.nahc.org/

ABOUT THE CONTRIBUTOR:

Shawn D'Amelio is director of business development at With a Little Help, Inc. and president of Washington Home Care Association. She may be reached at 206-352-7399. www.WithaLittleHelp.com.

CHAPTER 19

HEALTH CARE PROXY: APPOINTING SOMEONE TO MAKE YOUR MEDICAL DECISIONS

Who would you trust to make medical decisions for you if you are not able to make them yourself?

When working in the field of health advocacy, Beth Droppert, RN, BSN and I often came across people who lived alone and needed someone to be appointed as medical decision-maker in case they were no longer able to make those decisions. When we were actively running our health advocacy business, we decided to offer the service as healthcare proxy to a select few people. It seemed so critically important for people who either had no family or close friends or did not want their family to be tasked with this important role.

A healthcare proxy (also referred to as a durable power of attorney for healthcare) is a document that appoints someone to make medical decisions for you if you are in a situation where you can't make them yourself. You must choose your proxy thoughtfully since he or she will be acting on your behalf. Without a healthcare proxy, a doctor may be required to provide you with medical treatment that you would have refused if you were able to do so.

One of the clients whom we worked with, Bea, was a long-time army nurse who had lived an exciting life living all over the world. Divorced for many years and in her early 70s, she was a highly intelligent, engaging woman who now lived alone in an apartment south of Seattle. She was a planner and had hired a financial fiduciary (responsible for her bill-paying) and had an estate planner who kept her legal affairs in order. But she didn't have any living family to serve the role of healthcare proxy. Beth and I took on that role, and also included another nurse as a back-up so we could be sure that one of the three of us knew Bea well and could respond should anything happen.

The healthcare proxy role is also called a healthcare decision surrogate. It is not a common role, and with the growing baby boomer population who have no children, it is sure to become more popular. But finding a health care proxy may be challenging in the near-term.

Julie Forkasdi is a geriatric care manager based in Seattle. She began her career learning advocacy in her work as a social worker in a guardianship agency. A guardian is a court-appointed licensed professional who oversees the care of someone who is incapacitated. Typically, this encompasses all aspects of care (including living arrangements, healthcare, financial affairs, etc.). Julie worked for a guardianship agency with clients who needed healthcare navigation assistance, and after 15 years she started her care management business, where she primarily works with aging adults.

Her typical clients are aging with some kind of dementia, and they want help with care management (navigating healthcare and coordination of companions who can assist with activities of daily living). Some of them also need a healthcare proxy, designated through a document called a power of attorney for healthcare.

Julie shared a recent story about a client of hers in her 60s who ten years ago had a brain aneurism and stroke that left her paralyzed on one side of her body. Roberta cannot see well and needs help with activities of daily living like cooking, personal care issues, cleaning and walking.

Roberta's ex-boyfriend served as an excellent advocate and made sure she was well situated in an assisted living home, with good companion care. He also identified and helped Roberta hire Julie to be the medical decision maker. Although less common, it has been helpful to have someone looking after the medical aspects of Roberta's care. For instance, Roberta hurt her leg and worried that something was wrong. Julie accompanied Roberta to the doctor to help communicate her health history and to advocate for her care moving forward. The doctor checked for a blood clot, which is common after a stroke and could be life-threatening.

For a different client, Ruth, who was in her 90s and had increasingly advanced dementia, Julie served as power of attorney for healthcare. Although Ruth had family, she wanted to have Julie be the healthcare proxy to avoid conflicts with family members and for peace of mind that Julie would follow her stated advance directives that outlined her wishes, including no tube feeding, and a do not resuscitate directive.

Ruth was living in a facility when she contracted pneumonia. Julie accompanied her to the hospital and despite receiving appropriate care, Ruth continued to decline. In speaking with the doctor and consulting Ruth's advance directive, Julie believed that hospice should be initiated. Julie spoke with the doctor, who was very young, about the options and asked him to have a consultation with the family to bring up and make a referral to hospice. The young doctor outlined all the treatment options, including those that Julie knew Ruth didn't want, including tube feeding. But when it came to the hospice option, the doctor froze and could not effectively discuss it. Julie chimed in, and the hospice referral was made, even though the family was unsure if the timing was right.

Hospice provides extra support, including nursing oversight, pain management, bathing assistance, and spiritual care. This support can be critically important in the home, as well as in a facility that might not have adequate staff to increase care. Five days after hospice was initiated, Ruth died. The family was grateful to have had that extra support.

Whether you select a family member, friend or independent healthcare proxy, you will want to consider if the person:

- is someone you can trust
- can make decisions that you would want, regardless of their personal opinions
- is available and responsive when you need it
- is geographically able to respond quickly
- has specific expertise (like a medical background) that could be helpful in medical decision-making
- is able to avoid family conflicts
- will be an effective communicator with health professionals

WHY IT MATTERS:

- A growing number of baby boomers are unmarried and childless, leaving a good portion of the population needing support for medical decision-making assistance.
- Treatments for which there is little to no benefit at end of life are common in the hospital and should be reviewed by the medical decision-maker.
- If you wait to assign a healthcare proxy and are unexpectedly injured, you might not have your ideal team of people helping you in the way you want.

USING THIS INFORMATION:

1. Select someone you trust to serve as your healthcare decision-maker and name her or him in your durable power of attorney document for healthcare. This document accompanies your will. Without it, you could receive treatment that you do not want.

2. If you want to use a non-family or friend, you can find people who serve as healthcare proxy by contacting health advocates, aging life care managers, or guardian agencies in your state. Not all of these people provide this service, so you have to ask.

3. Some considerations when hiring a healthcare proxy:

   - Can you contact the healthcare proxy 24 hours a day, 7 days a week either for emergency or non-emergency support?

   - If you are contracting with a company, ask if there is a specific person who will be your main decision-maker. Will there be a back-up?

   - If you are hiring an individual, ask what the plan is for when they are traveling or taking personal time.

   - How will the healthcare proxy understand what your wishes are? Are there a series of meetings over time? What is written down about your wishes and potential choices? Who has access to that information?

   - How will the healthcare proxy work with your family?

4. How do you find a healthcare proxy? Here are some places to identify people who might perform this function:

   - Aging Life Care Association: www.aginglifecare.org

- National Guardianship Organization: https://www.guardianship.org/find-a-guardian/
- WASHAA Directory (Washington State): http://www.washaa.org/washaa-health-advocates-directory-325426.html#!directory/map

5. You might expect to pay either a flat fee or ongoing fees to access a healthcare proxy. The fees can vary greatly. Make sure to ask how the fees are structured.

6. Always interview the person or people who will be responsible for decision-making on your behalf.

LANGUAGE YOU CAN USE:

- Will you (or your agency) be named in my power of attorney for healthcare?
- Will you take my call and be available to me 24 hours a day, 7 days a week? If not, what will happen if I need to be in touch with someone in an emergency?
- If you are unavailable, what will be our plan?
- Are there any wishes I have that you feel you could not support?
- What would you do if two healthcare professionals conflict in their advice?
- Have you been a healthcare proxy with other clients? If so, what was the most challenging part of the work?
- How do you charge for this work?
- If you no longer do this work in the future, do you have a plan for who will replace you?

ADDITIONAL READING AND RESOURCES:

- The costs of care at the end of life: https://www.debt.org/medical/hospice-costs/
- Honoring Choices: https://www.honoringchoicespnw.org/plan/talk-about-it/
- Useful online tool to discuss end of life planning: https://www.finalroadmap.com/

ABOUT THE CONTRIBUTOR:

Julie Forkasdi can be reached at julieforkasdi.com, julieforkasdi@gmail.com, or by phone at 206-948-1964.

CHAPTER 20

CONSIDER A DEATH DOULA

While many people recognize the role of a doula as a non-medical support coach for birth, the concept of a death doula is relatively new. According to Crystal Flores, a Seattle-area death doula, who calls herself a "death coach," this role complements hospice care for families who want to actively participate in and support their loved one through the dying process. The National End-of-Life Doula Alliance defines this role in the following way: End-of-life doulas provide non-medical, holistic support and comfort to the dying person and their family, which may include education and guidance as well as emotional, spiritual or practical care, from as early as initial diagnosis through bereavement.

Similar to hiring a birth doula to help you develop and follow a birth plan, death doulas are typically hired to help the dying person and his or her family through the labor of death by normalizing the process. Also, the doula can help the dying person create a legacy project, which helps them review and explore the meaning of their life.

Doulagivers™ Certified End of Life Doula Training teaches the four phases encountered at the end of life. It is helpful for families to know some information about the basic stages of the dying process:

- **Shock Phase:** The dying person has received a terminal diagnosis. Sometimes if this is a young person or a tragic accident, the family might not ever leave this stage.

- **Stabilization Phase:** The person has come to terms with their terminal diagnosis. This can be the most beautiful phase, because the person is generally lucid, can create a legacy project, have conversations surrounding forgiveness, or wrap up unresolved issues in relationships.

- **Transition Phase:** The dying person goes into a deep sleep and could be sleeping most of the time. When he or she is not sleeping, they may still be somewhat lucid. Conversations can happen, but they are generally short, so not much can be accomplished during this time.

- **Active Dying Phase:** This last stage of dying is when the body shuts down. The person is not really coherent, and if they appear to be awake, they might not be responsive. They might have a sort of glazed over look in their eyes, almost as if they are looking through you or they may keep their eyes closed the majority of the time.

Crystal recommends that people create a Death Intention, which is basically a plan for the dying process, a goal in words and images showcasing what is most sacred, meaningful, and important to them. This is a gift to the loved ones who surround the dying person. It gives a clear snapshot of how to best honor their dying loved one. It's best to create a Death Intention before it's needed, while still healthy. Crystal offers this in a workshop format.

Crystal's personal experience with the deaths of her parents led her to create her business, which she says bridges the gap between medical necessities that hospice provides and holistic comfort. She says that the most valuable thing that doulas have is time. Hospice providers only have a certain amount of time that they can spend with the patient and for specific purposes. The doula is there for everything else. For instance, planning a vigil, planning a celebration of life, organizing photos, legacy work, spiritual support, errands, general tasking and sometimes the dying person simply needs someone to confess wrongdoings to (i.e. maybe they have another wife or family). The doula is in place to allow loved ones to be present in the way they always have been. This restores dignity to the dying person and sets the stage for a meaningful experience.

It was her own personal family situation which led Crystal to her death doula business. She was living in San Francisco in 2015, working in corporate sales, making a nice salary, and living comfortably when she received a call from her father, Corbett. Both of Crystal's parents were nurses, who took an early retirement at age 63 and moved to the coastal town of Newport, Oregon, their "sanctuary."

Unfortunately, her mother Marjorie had been misdiagnosed at the small town hospital, having gone to the emergency room countless times in eight weeks due to symptoms of nausea, vomiting, and dizziness. The hospital told Marjorie she had the flu, a bug, a virus, ear infection, and various minor illnesses without conducting a lot of tests. At her final ER visit, they did a CAT scan of her head, which revealed a mass. Without the equipment to properly diagnose, they immediately transported Marjorie to Corvallis, the nearest town which could deal with her medical situation. Within hours, Marjorie was diagnosed with a brain tumor and was scheduled for emergency surgery the following day.

Marjorie came through the surgery but was not the same person following the 7-hour procedure. Her formal diagnosis was primary diffuse large B-cell lymphoma of the central nervous system. This is a rare, aggressive tumor originating in the brain. This type of cancer has been estimated to account for only 1% of all lymphomas. The tumor was located in the cerebellum and was the size of a cherry. There is no protocol to treat this type of cancer. Marjorie's prognosis was three months. The grieving process began right away.

Crystal remembered that her parents (who described themselves as former hippies) were vocal about not wanting chemotherapy or anything artificial if given a terminal diagnosis. However, Marjorie, not wanting to face potentially dying quickly and leaving her husband of 30 years, opted to do experimental chemotherapy.

Crystal describes her parents as always in love and inseparable. The thought of losing his wife was unbearable to Corbett. Crystal decided to leave her family and career in San Francisco and move in with her father, to teach him how to live without her mom. But three weeks into the treatment, Crystal discovered Corbett had passed away in his bed. Tragically, Corbett wasn't sick, he was broken, his heart shattered. Crystal believes that her father left this earth so Marjorie could let go too, knowing the chemo wouldn't do anything for her.

Crystal was shocked by her dad's death, and hours later had to face telling her mother this news as she sat in her hospital bed. That day, she became Marjorie's power of attorney, arranged for hospice and took her home. Marjorie died eight weeks after her husband.

Crystal built her business around the gaps she found in experiencing the deaths of her parents. Through her experience as a 24-hour caregiver, she understood how exhausting and stressful caring for your loved one is at the end of life. People would ask how to help, but, Crystal said, although she was grateful for support, she could not articulate what she needed. There were days she didn't shower or eat because she was focused on giving care. In her business now, she has a menu of typical needs that people can choose. When a person is in crisis mode, they lack the ability to realize what basic needs are being missed.

Crystal admits that she did some things she thought *would* be helpful, but in hindsight were really hurtful. After her dad died, she rearranged the house and got rid of the bedroom furniture so she could set Marjorie up in the living room so she could be near her mom's hospice bed. However, the bedroom was where her parents spent a lot of their time together. She didn't realize this would be so sad for her mom, who wanted to sit in the bedroom as it previously was. Crystal did the best she could.

After her parents' deaths, Crystal went back to San Francisco and packed up her family, deciding to move to Seattle. They had no place to live, no job and no idea about what they would do next. She said she was heavy with emotion and wanted to run away from her grief.

Crystal began volunteering with hospice in 2016 and found that as a volunteer there were so many rules about what you couldn't do with the family that it left her feeling like she couldn't do and say what would be truly helpful. Knowing she was capable of so much more, she went on to get her doula certification through Doula-givers™ in addition to training through International End of Life Doula Association (INELDA) and founded her business in 2017.

Crystal's goal with her business is to prevent anybody else from feeling the brokenness and aloneness she felt at that time. Although she had to guess at how her parents would like to be honored, her work today helps families plan to do just that.

Today, there are many ways that death doulas, like Crystal work with clients. Crystal conducts a lot of workshops to educate and empower families. She typically works with just one family at a time and as an example will be in residence for three days and nights. This allows family members to give attention to their loved one without having to only perform the required caregiving tasks needed.

Instead of spending all of their time with a checklist of what has to be done, including administering medicines, the family gets to come and go and have meaningful conversations with their loved one. These conversations are what make a person feel human – the doula allows every family member to maintain their normal role with that person, instead of solely focusing on caregiving.

Crystal's role also focuses on facilitating conversation, and she often conducts a forgiveness ceremony. She identifies where the struggles were or are and what is unfinished business that would be helpful for the family to resolve. This creates a level of freedom for the person dying and allows loved ones to give and receive forgiveness.

Although not covered by insurance, families can expect to pay either hourly rates or a total amount of $500 or more, depending on their needs. Crystal said that the death doula movement is really shedding light on bringing death back to families and empowering them to do this in a way that is meaningful and dignified, the way we did it a century ago.

WHY IT MATTERS:

- Studies have shown that approximately 80% of Americans would prefer to die at home. Despite this, 60% of Americans die in acute care hospitals, 20% in nursing homes and only 20% at home.[61]

- 56% of people have not communicated their end-of life wishes, according to the Survey of Californians by the California HealthCare Foundation (2012).

- While 80% of people say that if seriously ill, they would want to talk to their doctor about wishes for medical treatment toward the end of their life, only 7% report having had this conversation with their doctor, according to the same survey.

---

[61] https://palliative.stanford.edu/home-hospice-home-care-of-the-dying-patient/where -do-americans-die/

- Two out of three adults living in the United States have not completed an advance directive, a document telling people what their wishes are for end of life.[62]

USING THIS INFORMATION:

1. Consider hiring a death doula or coach if you feel that would benefit your dying loved one.
2. You can find a death doula through one of the links at the INELDA at: https://www.inelda.org/ or Doula Givers at: https://www.doulagivers.com/find-a-doula/
3. Ask the death doula what options you have for utilizing their services.

SPECIFIC LANGUAGE YOU CAN USE WHEN INTERVIEWING A DEATH DOULA:

- What services can you provide my family?
- How do you charge for your services?
- How do you work with hospice?
- What is the difference between what you provide and the services of a normal caregiver?
- Are you bonded and insured?
- What have people found to be most valuable in utilizing your services?
- Do you have references and a background check?

---

[62] https://www.sciencedaily.com/releases/2017/07/170705184048.htm

ADDITIONAL READING AND RESOURCES:

- General overview article about doulas: https://www.psycholo gytoday.com/us/blog/understanding-grief/201805/doulas -the-dying
- Detailed article about doula roles, history, etc.: http://www. todaysgeriatricmedicine.com/archive/JF19p12.shtml
- There are two directories to find death doulas who go through a certification process:

  https://www.inelda.org/find-doula/

  https://www.doulagivers.com/find-a-doula/
- AARP article on death doulas: https://www.aarp.org/care-giving/home-care/info-2018/end-of-life-doulas.html
- Great article about why you may not want to die at home: https://www.theguardian.com/commentisfree/2017/may/ 01/dying-at-home-terminally-ill-hospital

ABOUT THE CONTRIBUTOR:

Crystal Flores is a death coach/doula whose business is Your Ultimate Love Story https://www.yourultimatelovestory.com/

To contact Robin about speaking at your event, community, or to inquire about creative consulting for your organization, visit:

www.Robin-Shapiro.Com

Follow Robin at

@WellSaidHealth   @AHAAdvocate   @WellSaidHealth

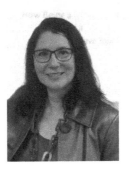

BOOK CLUB DISCUSSION QUESTIONS

Q. What story from this book is unforgettable to you? Why?

Q. This book focuses on actions you can take. Are there any suggested actions that you plan to do? If so, when?

Q. Where do you keep your medical and health wishes in writing?

Q. Do you have someone, or more than one person who you can count on to be your advocate if you need one?

- How did you pick that person?

- Do you think they will be the best person to support you when making medical decisions? Why or why not?

- If you don't have an advocate, what is your plan for identifying and talking with someone?

Q. After reading this book, do you think you would make a good health advocate for a family member or friend? Why or why not?

Q. Do you have a good relationship with your primary care doctor? If you could change one thing, what would it be?

Q. If your medical story was highlighted with a topic for this book, what would it be?

Q. What topics do you wish were covered in the book but weren't?

AUTHOR'S BIO

Robin Shapiro is a successful entrepreneur and nationally recognized expert and pioneer in the health advocacy field. She has spent her 30+ year career helping patients find their voice to improve their care. She has founded award-winning businesses that focus on empowering patients by utilizing their personal stories and identifying what matters most ... to ultimately lead to better health. She is currently the Board Chair of WASHAA, the Washington State Health Advocacy Association, whose mission is to help people transform from patient to active participant and partner in their health. She lives in Seattle with her husband and two dogs, Lucky and Butters.

CPSIA information can be obtained
at www.ICGtesting.com
Printed in the USA
LVHW031357260121
677404LV00004B/171

9 781087 809069